A Manual for Designing Your Own Practice

YOGA FOR THE WEST . . .

"emphasizes the fact that time, culture, society, food, and genetic factors cannot be discarded when one wants to look at yoga with the intention of reducing problems and promoting health and well-being."

— *Desikachar*

At last, a book has been written by an experienced Westerner for Westerners that applies the ancient principles of yoga to the modern person's needs — by concentrating on an *individualized* approach. By utilizing modifications of traditional postures that specifically suit himself or herself, the modern yoga practitioner can systematically develop a program that is infinitely flexible and personally appropriate.

YOGA FOR THE WEST

YOGA FOR THE WEST

A manual for designing your own practice.

Ian Rawlinson

Edited by Alastair McNeilage

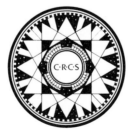

CRCS PUBLICATIONS
Post Office Box 1460
Sebastopol, California 95472

Library of Congress Cataloging in Publication Data

Rawlinson, Ian, 1947–
    Yoga for the West.

    1. Yoga, Hatha.   I. Title.
RA781.7.R38   1985   613.7'046   85-13235
ISBN 0-916360-26-1 (pbk.)

First Edition
INTERNATIONAL STANDARD BOOK NUMBER (ISBN): 0-916360-26-1
First published in the USA by CRCS Publications
Published simultaneously in Great Britain by Unwin Paperbacks, an imprint of Unwin Hyman Ltd.
PUBLISHER'S NOTE: Readers of this book should take the advice contained herein to find an appropriate teacher for their yogic practice, which will go a long way toward enabling them to make the most from this book without any harmful side-effects. The publisher takes no responsibility for any misunderstandings or alleged harmful results from anyone's actions based upon, or alleged to be based upon, the instructions in this volume. Any severe physical or psychological problem should be referred to a professional practitioner whose expertise is appropriate for the problem.

This book is dedicated to
Desikachar
with whom it has been my
good fortune to study.

Contents

Acknowledgements

I would like to express my deep sense of gratitude to Desikachar for the help he gave me in writing this book. Without his help, it would not have been possible. He made invaluable suggestions as to its form, answered hundreds of my questions, and checked the manuscript.

Alastair McNeilage's help has also been of immense value. As an experienced writer he was able to edit the book thoroughly and make suggestions where passages needed clarification and rewriting. Without his help I doubt if the book would have been completed.

Roland Short of the Cambridge Camera Club has been extremely generous with his time and expertise in taking the photographs. My thanks also to Karen Melvin for taking the photograph for the cover.

I would also like to thank my pupils and friends who helped in so many ways, particularly Woods Shoemaker, Maureen Tobias and Su Prynne for their encouragement. To Naomi Dale and Michael Meadway, my thanks for acting as models for the photographs, and to Christina Clough and Tina Bone for typing the manuscript.

Last but not least I would like to thank my parents, my parents-in-law and my wife for their support.

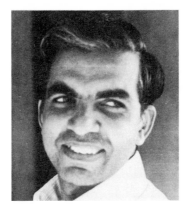

Foreword

When I began taking a serious look at yoga in 1963, yoga was a curiosity for everyone around me. But the situation today is very different. In different ways yoga has entered into the life of millions everywhere. In fact more information on yoga is available today than, say, on ecology.

This has created a situation where people expect a little more than curiosity value from a book on yoga. They expect a valid, scientifically acceptable exposition. The texts which tell one what to do on Monday, what is the appropriate yoga for asthma, etc. (irrespective of whether or not you are also suffering from, say, back pain or you are pregnant), are being seriously questioned. Ian Rawlinson's attempt is here before you; an attempt at explaining the What, When, How and Why of Asana and Pranayama. His hard work, of course, has limitations. No text can replace direct oral transmission when it talks about the body and the mind, which are always in a state of flux. But I believe that the attempt is an eye-opener. It emphasises the fact that time, culture, society, food and genetic factors cannot be discarded when one wants to look at yoga with the intention of reducing problems and promoting health and well-being.

DESIKACHAR

Introduction

In the early 1970s, after I had been practising yoga for seven years, I was fortunate to have a lesson from a teacher who had studied with Desikachar. The approach was totally different from any system I had come across up to that time. While I was familiar with some techniques of practising yoga postures and breathing techniques, many aspects of Desikachar's approach were new, particularly the extensive use of modifying postures and the great precision in the way the breath was used in the postures. What also really excited me about the approach was the way the practice was adapted to the individual. This was particularly noticeable in the way the asanas were arranged into a sequence or Vinyasa. I found that when the sequence was adapted to my needs, choosing variations, modifications and a sequence of postures which would help prepare for the main posture of the Vinyasa, the quality of my practice was greatly improved. I was immediately interested in studying the approach in more depth and wrote to Desikachar asking for permission to study with him in India.

I spent the following winter with him in Madras. Desikachar teaches in the traditional way, taking a small number of students at a time and working with them primarily in individual classes. Several times a week I would cycle over to his house in the suburbs of Madras for my classes. Gradually over the months he explained the theoretical and practical aspects of practising asanas and pranayama.

The first principle Desikachar explained in detail was Vinyasa — how to arrange a sequence of postures in an intelligent order, so that there is a goal; preparation for the goal; and a gradual descent after the goal has been reached. This principle is very highly developed in this tradition and lays a great deal of emphasis on adapting the practice according to the individual. He explained that the sequence, or Vinyasa, that is helpful to one person may not be helpful to another — in fact it could be detrimental.

The more I examined this concept, of yoga practice tailored to the individual, the more sense it made. Teaching everyone in the same way seemed to me rather like expecting everyone to wear size ten shoes.

As my classes progressed we examined other aspects of this tradition, particularly the very precise way in which the breath can be used in the postures. Again, when this principle is adapted to the individual, it adds an immensely beneficial dimension to the practice. Up until this time my use of breath had been rather haphazard, but with a clear explanation of the basic principles it took on a much greater depth and significance.

We also examined the use of modifications and variations to adapt the practice to the individual. Desikachar explained that by intelligently selecting a variation or modification, the practice could be made much more effective. He showed how, simply by bending the knees a little in a forward-bending asana, the *quality* of the pose could be improved.

Gradually as the months went by the different principles became integrated into my own practice. The purpose of this book is to describe those principles of practising asana and pranayama as taught to me by Desikachar.

In India, great importance has always been placed on direct tuition, and Desikachar himself continues this tradition. The written word cannot be a substitute for personal teaching, but it can help on a theoretical level. For a practical application of the principles described, personal tuition is, in my opinion, essential.

Ian Rawlinson
PO Box 2952
Petaluma
California 94952
USA

YOGA FOR
THE WEST

CHAPTER 1

Vinyasa in Asana

Vinyasa is vitally important to the practice of asanas. It encourages a creative attitude to your approach to yoga and enables you to plan and structure your practice, changing and adapting it according to your needs.

The word itself means 'to begin at a particular point, gradually ascend to a set goal and then descend again' *(see Fig. 1.1)*. When applied to the practice of asanas, it entails the selection of a number of postures arranged in an intelligent sequence with a definite aim. Your goal could be a particular posture, or it might be to hold a position for a certain length of time, or again, it could be to use a breathing ratio in a number of asanas — there are many possibilities. In Vinyasa some postures will be used to prepare for the main purpose of the practice, others as a gradual descent, for, in the words of Vamadeva, 'without recourse to Vinyasa asanas cannot be mastered'.

Vinyasa is important both psychologically and physiologically. The psychological importance lies in preparing a sequence of asanas so that there is a definite structure and shape, thus making it easier for the mind to concentrate.

The physiological importance of Vinyasa is obvious. If you attempt asanas, particularly the more strenuous ones, without adequate preparation, you may well injure yourself. For example, if the first posture in a practice is a strong back bend such as Urdhva

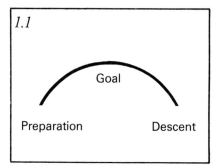

1.1

Goal

Preparation   Descent

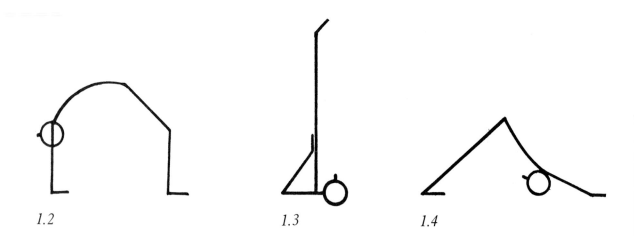

1.2   *1.3*   *1.4*

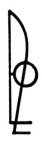

1.5

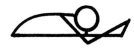

1.6

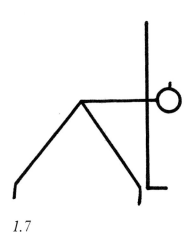

1.7

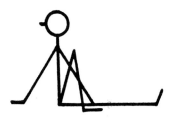

1.8

Dhanurasana *(Fig. 1.2)*, without any preparation you can severely damage your back and shoulders.

If your body is prepared, you can improve the quality of the main posture and hold it for longer. An example of this is Sarvangasana *(Fig. 1.3)*. For example, some people find that if Adhomukha Svanasana *(Fig. 1.4)* is done first, they can hold Sarvangasana much longer because they have already well prepared the head in an inverted position. There are many other instances where correct preparation improves the quality of the main pose.

Usually a particular asana (or asanas) can be selected as the main aim of the practice. Often this will be the most demanding asana in a sequence, and the one which affects particular areas of the body most vigorously — areas which need to be thoroughly prepared beforehand.

It should be stressed that the preparation and descent within a Vinyasa will vary a great deal according to your own physical condition.

General sequence of asanas

There are no absolute rules in the practice of asanas and their order. The order varies according to the mental and physical make-up of each individual and the length of time each person has been practising yoga.

However, the following sequences of asanas will help to illustrate the basic idea:

1 Standing
2 Lying
3 Inverted
4 Back bend
5 Twisting
6 Forward bend

In general, the first posture of a Vinyasa should be a simple forward-bend, because the body is more used to this type of movement. Twisting and back-bending postures should only be introduced once the body has warmed up.

Standing postures

Standing postures are the most effective way of warming up the body and usually come at the beginning of the sequence. The first few postures are generally practised dynamically, i.e. each posture is repeated (see Chapter 4) in order to warm and remove stiffness. This is important when practising in the morning. Certain standing postures are especially useful in acting as preparation for a main asana or asanas. A standing forward-bend such as Uttanasana *(Fig. 1.5)* is helpful as a preparation for Pascimatanasana *(Fig. 1.6)*. Similarly, the standing twisting posture, Trikonasana *(Fig. 1.7)* prepares for Ardha Matsyendrasana *(Fig. 1.8)*.

15

Lying postures

Lying postures come after standing postures and prepare for the inverted asanas. Urdhva Prasrta Padasana *(Fig. 1.9)*, for example, prepares the legs and stomach muscles for going up into Sarvangasana *(Fig. 1.10)*. Dvipada Pitham *(Fig. 1.11)* prepares the neck for Sarvangasana. Lying postures also give you a chance to recuperate after standing postures and act as an intermediate stage between standing and inverted asanas.

Inverted postures

Inverted postures usually come in the middle of the Vinyasa. The standing and lying postures have thoroughly prepared all those areas of the body you will be using when you go up into the inverted postures. Usually, Sirsasana *(Fig. 1.12)* comes first and is followed by Sarvangasana which acts as a counter-pose for the neck.

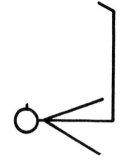

1.9

Back-bending postures

After Sarvangasana a back-bending movement is necessary to counteract the strong effects on the neck and shoulders. Bhujangasana *(Fig. 1.13)* or Salabhasana *(Fig. 1.14)* are both suitable. They also act as preparation for the more strenuous back bends such as Ustrasana *(Fig. 1.15)* and Urdhva Dhanurasana *(Fig. 1.16)*.

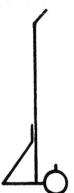

1.10

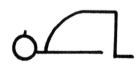

1.11

1.12

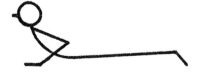

1.13

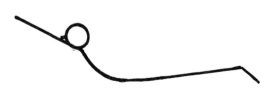

1.14

Twisting postures

Twisting postures such as Ardha Matsyendrasana *(Fig. 1.17)* come in between back bends and forward bends. Back bends work vigorously on the back and are often useful preparation for twisting. Since twisting postures themselves help to loosen the hips and prepare for forward bends, they are particularly helpful if you have stiff hips.

Forward-bending postures

Forward-bending postures such as Vajrasana *(Fig. 1.18),* or Pascimatanasana *(Fig. 1.19)* follow twists, acting as a counter-pose as they help to realign the muscles and organs of the body. They also help to lengthen the breath, which will have become shorter during the twisting postures. This is important if you plan to follow your practice with Pranayama.

Resumé

To sum up, *Fig. 1.20* shows a Vinyasa which includes all types of postures. Standing, lying, inverted, back bends, twists and forward bends follow each other in a well-planned sequence of preparation and counter-pose (see Chapter 2).

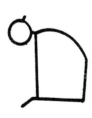

1.15

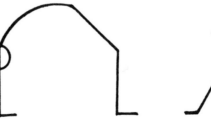

1.16

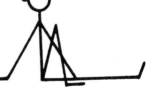

1.17

1.18

1.19

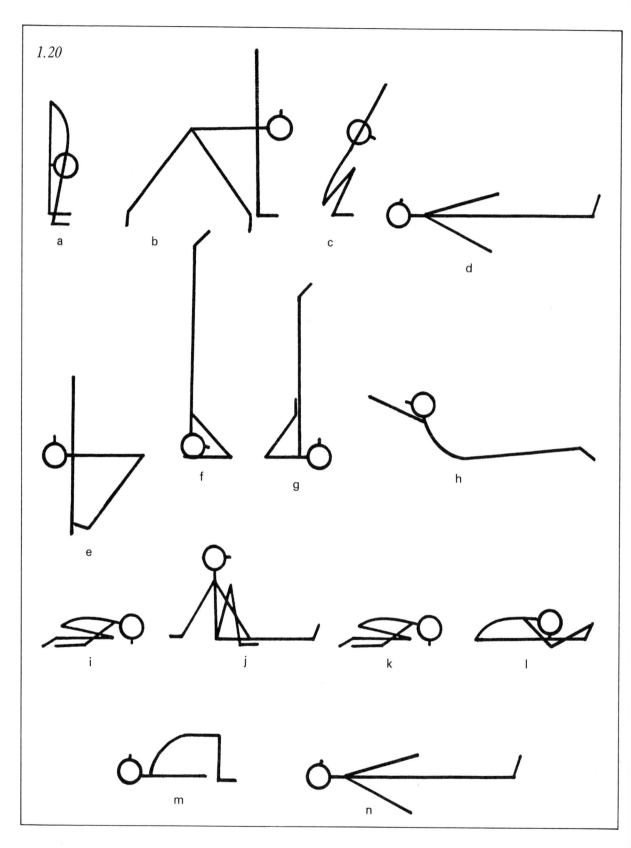

1.20

a

b

c

d

e

f

g

h

i

j

k

l

m

n

Examples of Vinyasa

A Vinyasa need not include all the types of asanas; you simply may not have time for such a long practice. It could merely consist of standing, lying and forward bends *(Fig. 1.21)*.

Figure 1.21i is, strictly speaking, out of sequence but acts as a valuable counter-posture to two forward-bending asanas.

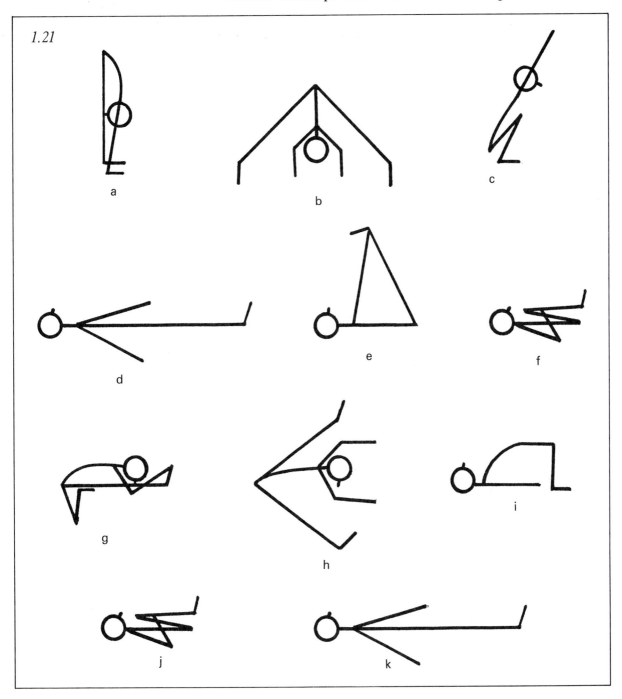

1.21

a

b

c

d

e

f

g

h

i

j

k

Figure 1.22 is another example of a shorter practice consisting of standing, lying, twisting and forward bends.

The general sequence can be taken out of order to suit your particular needs. In Figure 1.23 the lying postures act as preparation for the standing postures. They are useful for older students or if you are returning to yoga after illness or childbirth, as are sitting, standing back-bend and forward-bend postures (Figure 1.24 is an example). In this case beginning with sitting postures is helpful if you have very loose hips and consequently find postures such as Uttanasana and Parsva Uttanasana *(Fig. 1.25a and b)* too easy.

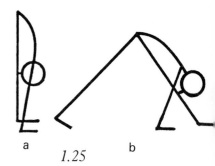

1.25

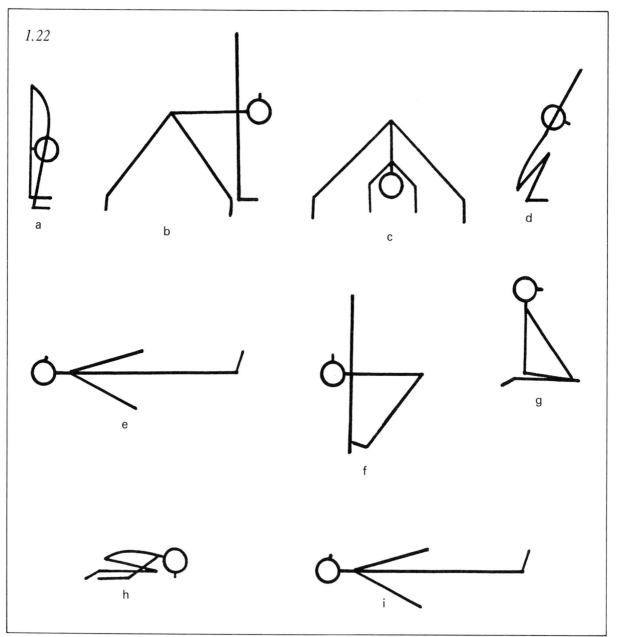

1.22

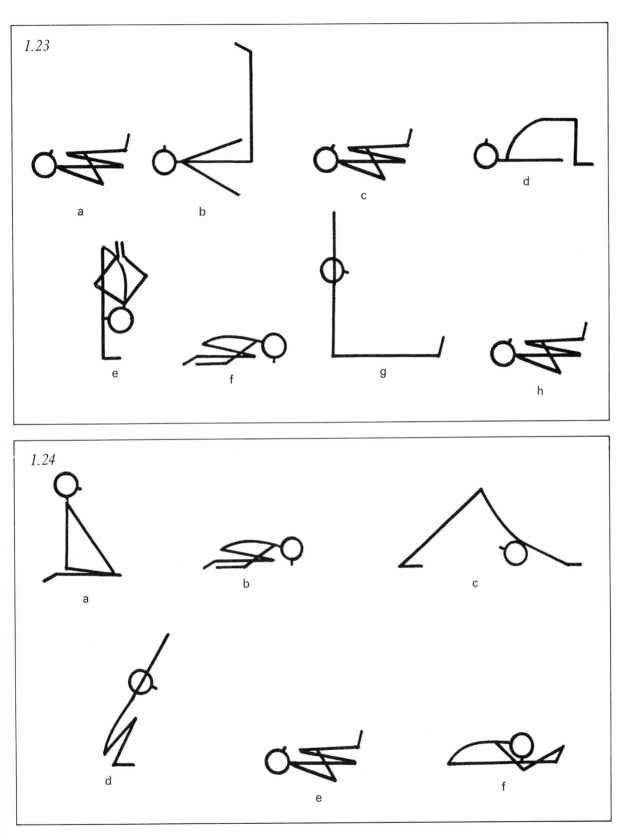

1.23

a

b

c

d

e

f

g

h

1.24

a

b

c

d

e

f

21

You can prepare for the same posture in a number of ways. The following are different Vinyasas for Sirsasana *(Fig. 1.26i)*. The first example *(Fig. 1.26)* prepares the shoulders and neck in particular. The next example *(Fig. 1.27)* includes Trikonasana (b) and Jathara Parivrtti (f), which often help correct twisting in the main pose.

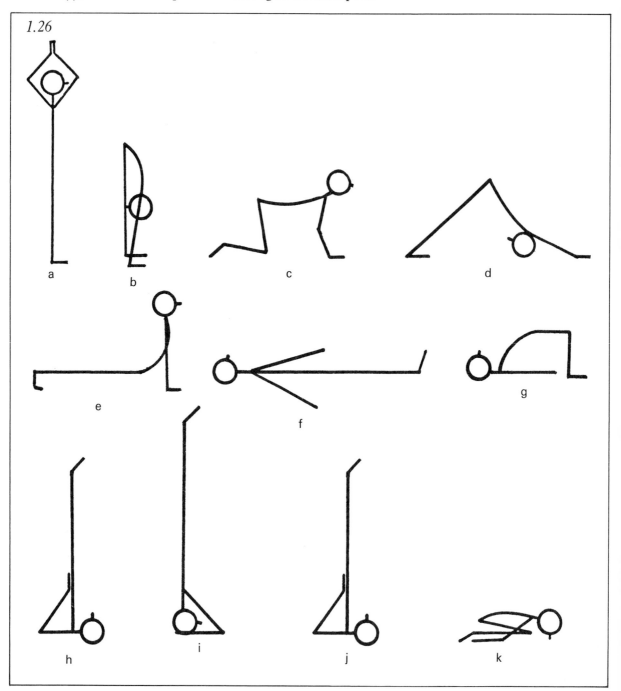

1.26

a

b

c

d

e

f

g

h

i

j

k

1.27

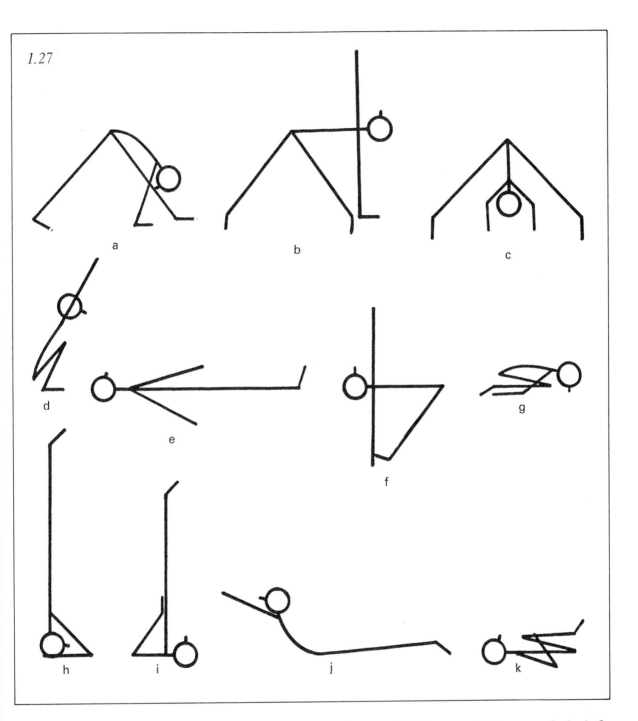

There are many other possible Vinyasas which prepare the body for Sirsasana. The choice depends upon you and your individual needs but usually each Vinyasa should contain a definite goal.

Vinyasa and variations

Variations of postures are often useful in preparation for the main pose, especially when the main pose is itself a variation. For example, if Ekapada Urdhva Dhanurasana *(Fig. 1.28)* is the main posture, the variations in Fig. 1.29 would be useful as preparation for the legs, hips and lower back, while variations of Ardha Padmasana *(Fig. 1.30)* can be used to help prepare for Padmasana *(Fig. 1.31)*. (You should have the guidance of a teacher before attempting Padmasana.)

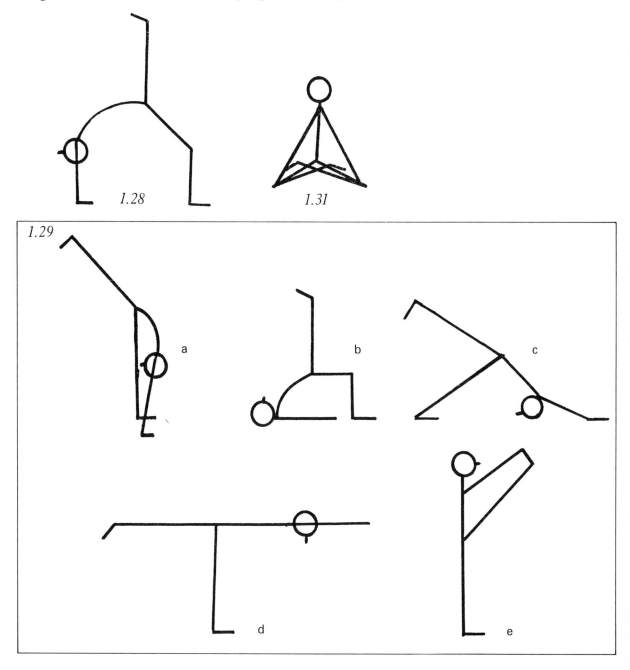

1.28

1.31

1.29

a

b

c

d

e

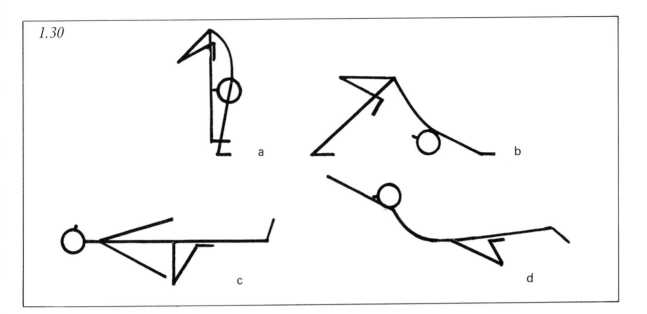

1.30

You don't always need to have a main posture within a Vinyasa. Your practice might be very simple, consisting of postures of the same intensity *(Fig. 1.32)*. This is useful when you are just starting to practise asanas, when you are very tired or when beginning to practise after an illness.

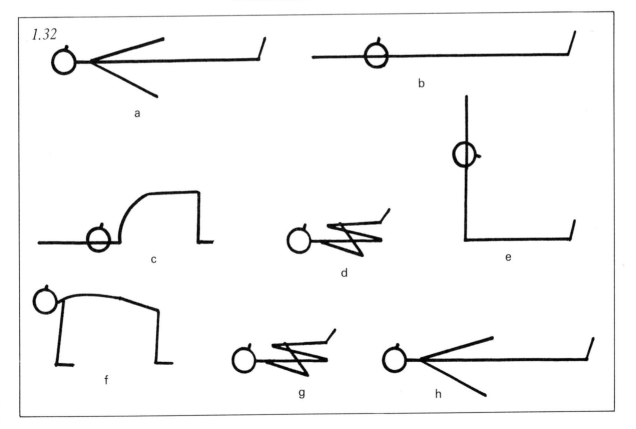

1.32

Combinations of Vinyasa

The previous examples show there is a considerable amount of variety in the ways a Vinyasa can be planned. Some of the main combinations are summarised for you below.

1 a Standing
    b Lying
    c Inverted
    d Back bend
    e Twist
    f Forward bend
    g Other sitting posture

2 a Lying
    b Standing
    c Forward bend
    d Sitting posture

3 a Standing
    b Lying
    c Forward bend

4 a Sitting
    b Standing
    c Back bend
    d Forward bend

5 a Lying
    b Sitting
    c Lying

6 a Standing
    b Lying
    c Forward bend

The principle of Vinyasa also applies within a particular group of asanas, with less demanding postures acting as a preparation for the more vigorous postures in the same group. In the back-bend group you can use Dhanurasana *(Fig. 1.33)* and Ekapada Ustrasana *(Fig. 1.34)* to prepare for Kapotasana *(Fig. 1.35)*.

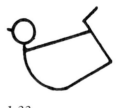

1.33

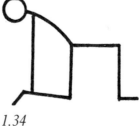

1.34

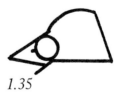

1.35

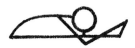

1.36

In the forward-bend group you could use Pascimatanasana *(Fig. 1.36)* and Janu Sirsasana *(Fig. 1.37)* to prepare for Upavista Konasana *(Fig. 1.38)*.

The principle of Vinyasa also applies when learning postures. Simpler postures need to be mastered before attempting harder ones. So, before you attempt Sirsasana *(Fig. 1.39)* you should be able to hold Sarvangasana *(Fig. 1.40)* comfortably for 5—10 minutes, and you should also be proficient in the postures in Fig. 1.41.

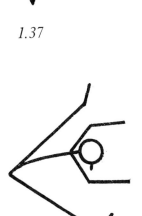

1.37

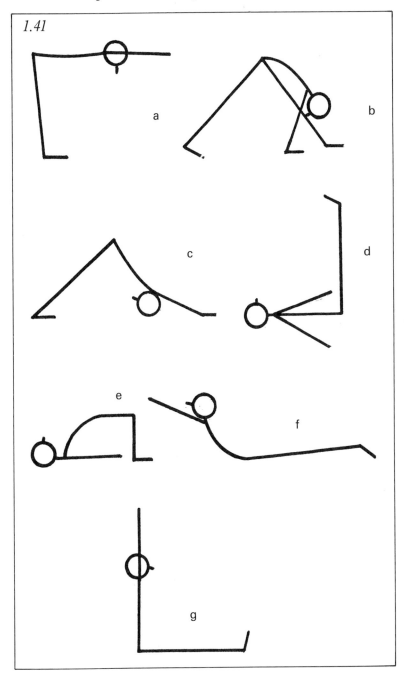

1.41

a

b

c

d

e

f

g

1.38

1.39   1.40

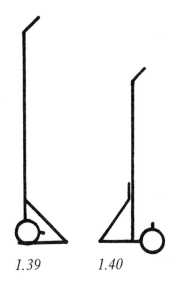

Similarly you should not attempt strong back-bends such as Viparita Dandasana *(Fig. 1.42)* without first mastering Ustrasana *(Fig. 1.43a)*, Dhanurasana *(Fig. 1.43b)* and Urdhva Dhanurasana *(Fig. 1.43c)*.

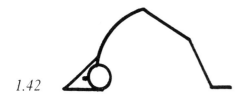

1.42

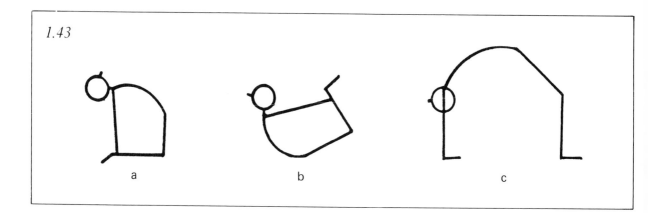

1.43

a   b   c

If your body is stiff or weak, you may find the full posture is not possible and to begin with the movement into the posture needs to be limited. In Pascimatanasana *(Fig. 1.44)* you could stop the movement when your back begins to bend. *It is far more beneficial to move halfway into a posture properly than to complete the movement badly.* When your body becomes more supple you can gradually increase the movement forward.

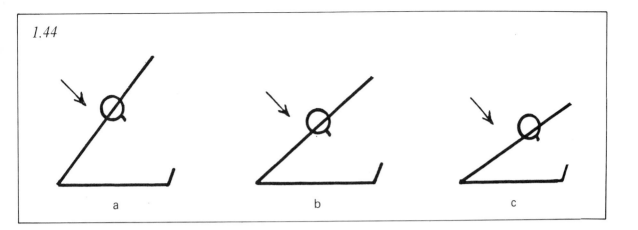

1.44

a   b   c

Changing a Vinyasa

You can gradually change a Vinyasa over a period of several days. One or two postures can be dropped and others introduced. This is best when first beginning to practise. As you become more familiar with postures and your body becomes suppler and stronger, changes from one type of Vinyasa to another can be done more easily and quickly.

Planning a Vinyasa

A number of factors will influence a Vinyasa:

1 Mental condition
2 Physical condition
3 Time of day
4 Time available for practice

You need to consider all these factors when deciding on your goal. For example, if your mind is dull and heavy, why not choose a stimulating practice to make you feel alert? Similarly, someone with a very stiff body will need to plan a different Vinyasa to someone with a very supple body.

The time of day makes a considerable difference to a Vinyasa. In the morning, when your body is stiff, you will need to spend time and care on planning the first part of a Vinyasa in order to ensure that the stiffness is removed. Standing postures are particularly helpful in such a situation. In contrast, when practising later in the day, especially if you have already practised in the morning, your preparation need not be for so long. However, a very stimulating evening practice will probably make sleeping difficult.

To sum up, you first of all need to choose a particular goal as the aim of the practice. This could be:

1 an asana, or asanas, such as a strong back-bend or an equally vigorous posture;
2 to see how long a particular posture can be held;
3 to see how a posture is affected by a particular breathing ratio;
4 to determine the longest breathing ratio possible in a particular asana or asanas.

Having decided upon the aim, spend some time planning how the practice should be arranged. It is often helpful to jot down beforehand the sequence, with the number of breaths or breathing ratios you intend to try in each posture. Make sure that the three aspects of Vinyasa — preparation, goal and descent — are included in the practice.

The previous pages outline the main aspects of Vinyasa. It should be emphasised that to employ these principles effectively, you need the advice and help of an experienced teacher who can modify the practice according to your individual needs.

Questions and observations

1 What comments can you make about the sequence in Fig. 1.45?
2 Prepare four Vinyasas for yourself, two for a morning practice and two for an evening practice.
3 Arrange the asanas in Fig. 1.46 into a Vinyasa.
4 Prepare a Vinyasa, lasting thirty minutes, which would be particularly useful in obtaining a relaxed state of mind.

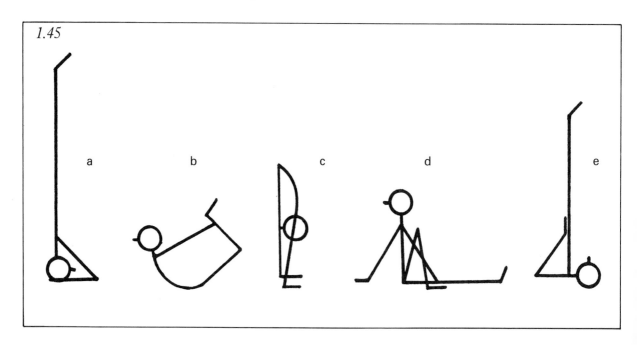

1.45

a   b   c   d   e

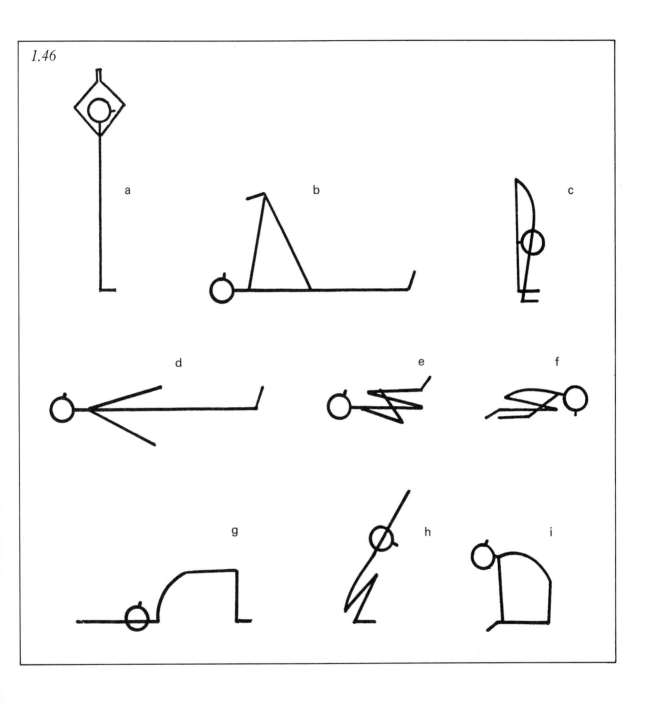

a

b

c

d

e

f

g

h

i

CHAPTER 2

The Principles of the Counter-pose

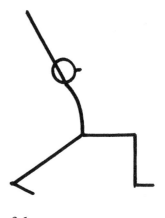

2.1

A counter-pose removes the negative effects of previous asanas and so helps you maintain a psychological balance during your practice. Usually a counter-pose works in the opposite direction to the previous asana, but in a gentler, less vigorous way.

The psychological and physiological need for a counter-pose

Psychological balance

In order to decide what would be a suitable counter-pose you need to observe the mental and physical effects of the previous asana or asanas. Let us first consider the mental effects. With dynamic, vigorous, expanding postures such as Virabhadrasana *(Fig. 2.1)*, Trikonasana *(Fig. 2.2)* and Ustrasana *(Fig. 2.3)*, the psychological effect is one of opening and releasing mental inhibitions and tensions. In order to keep these effects in balance it is necessary to counteract these postures with contracting movements such as Uttanasana *(Fig. 2.4)* or Vajrasana *(Fig. 2.5)*.

Conversely, strong forward-bending postures, such as Pascimatanasana *(Fig. 2.6)*, need expanding counter-postures such as Dvipada Pitham *(Fig. 2.7)*, or Cakravakasana *(Fig. 2.8)*, to maintain a psychological balance.

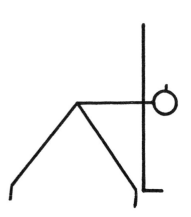

2.2

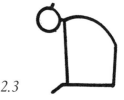

2.3

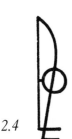

2.4

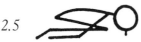

2.5

2.6

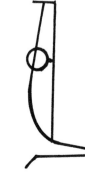

2.7

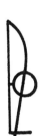

2.8

Physiological balance

In order to balance the physical effects of the previous asana or asanas, you should observe which parts of the body have been worked the most and will therefore need compensation. Some examples will help to illustrate this point.

With a vigorous asana such as Uttanasana *(Fig. 2.9)* the muscles in the back and the hamstrings in the backs of the legs are stretched quite vigorously and the opposite movement, in which they are contracted (for example, Utkatasana *(Fig. 2.10)* or Apanasana *(Fig. 2.11))*, helps counteract this stretching.

In a sitting posture such as Krauncasana *(Fig. 2.12)* the back and legs are also stretched and the chest is compressed. A counter-pose such as Dvipada Pitham *(Fig. 2.7)* removes the negative effects by opening the chest and back muscles, loosening the shoulders and bending the legs.

Sirsasana *(Fig. 2.13)* is a posture for which the correct counter-pose is very important. In this asana a lot of weight will be on your neck. If, after the pose has been held, the neck is stretched after being compressed, then the negative effects are removed. In this case, Sarvangasana *(Fig. 2.14)* is a suitable counter-pose.

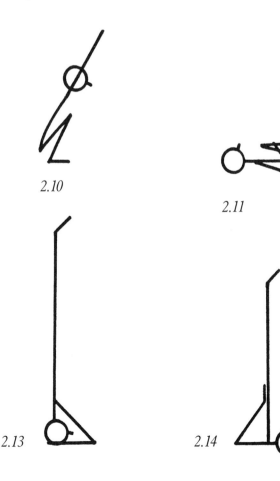

2.9

2.10

2.11

2.12

2.13

2.14

More than one counter-pose

One counter-pose may not be sufficient to remove the combined effects of an asana. Trikonasana *(Fig. 2.15)* is a posture which needs two counter-poses. As a twisting posture, it needs a forward bend as a counter-pose in order to help the muscles and organs realign themselves, so you could follow Trikonasana with Prasrta Pada Uttanasana *(Fig. 2.16)*. However, this in turn will need a counter-pose for the legs, hips and groin, and back, such as Utkatasana *(Fig. 2.17)*.

Another example of an asana that needs two counter-postures is a strong back-bend such as Ustrasana *(Fig. 2.18)*. After this asana you might find that a gentle forward-bend such as Vajrasana *(Fig. 2.19)* is not a strong enough counter-pose on its own and you may well need a stronger forward-bend such as Pascimatanasana *(Fig. 2.20)*.

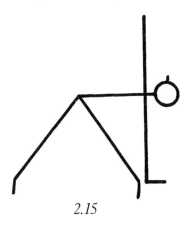

2.15

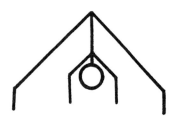

2.16

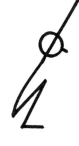

2.17

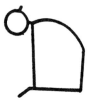

2.18

2.19

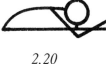

2.20

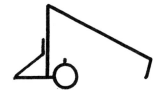

2.21

Dynamic and static use of counter-pose

Generally, if a posture has been held statically, the counter-pose should be dynamic. This helps in working on and loosening the areas which have undergone the greatest exertion. For example, if Viparita Dandasana *(Fig. 2.21)* has been held statically for several minutes, the counter-pose, Halasana *(Fig. 2.22)*, should be dynamic. Similarly, in Virasana *(Fig. 2.23)* the knees are rotated and then remain static; a dynamic counter-pose such as Apanasana *(Fig. 2.24a and b)* helps to free the joints.

2.22

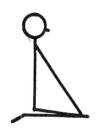

2.23

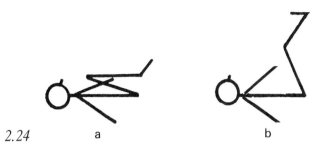

2.24   a   b

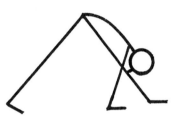

2.25

If, on the other hand, a posture such as Parsva Uttanasana *(Fig. 2.25)* or Prasrta Pada Uttanasana *(Fig. 2.26)* has been used dynamically, its counter-pose, Vajrasana *(Fig. 2.27)*, can be static. This is by no means a hard and fast rule, however; your strength, suppleness and quality of concentration will influence your choice of counter-pose, and what may be a suitable counter-pose for you may not suit someone else. For example, one counter-pose for Pascimatanasana *(Fig. 2.28)* is Purvatanasana *(Fig. 2.29)*. If, however, your hips are very stiff and their movement is limited, this asana will not be very effective and so Catuspadapitham *(Fig. 2.30)* or Dvipada Pitham *(Fig. 2.31)* would be better alternatives.

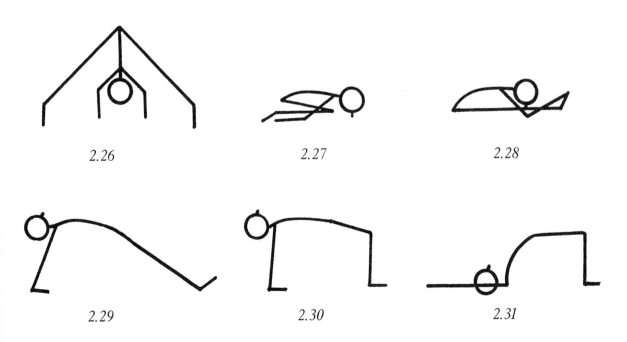

2.26   2.27   2.28

2.29   2.30   2.31

Similarly, although Pascimatanasana might be a
suitable counter-pose for the twisting posture, Maricyasana *(Fig. 2.32)*, you might find this too strenuous, in which case a gentler pose such as Vajrasana *(Fig. 2.33)* or Apanasana *(Fig. 2.34)* would be more suitable.

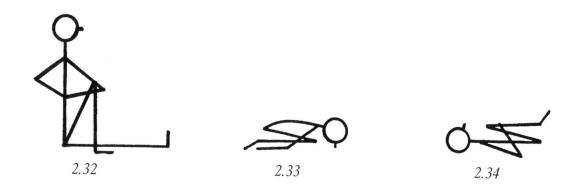

2.32   2.33   2.34

Length of counter-pose

How long you hold a counter-pose will vary according to how strenuous you find that particular posture. A general guide, however, is a third to a half of the total number of breaths taken during the previous asana or asanas.

Before attempting a new posture it is important that you make sure that you are capable of the counter-pose. Since most counter-poses are fairly easy postures, this is not usually a problem. However, Sirsasana *(Fig. 2.35)* is an exception; before attempting this posture you should be able to hold its counter-poses, Sarvangasana *(Fig. 2.36)*, Bhujanga-sana *(Fig. 2.37)* or Salabhasana *(Fig. 2.38)*.

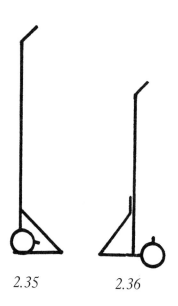

2.35   2.36

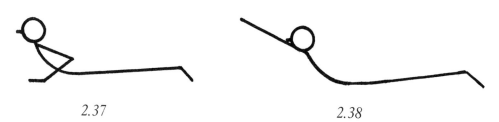

2.37   2.38

Savasana — an important counter-pose

Savasana *(Fig. 2.39)* is used as a counter-posture, both between different asanas or groups of asanas and sometimes following Pranayama. It is a very important posture and you should include it regularly during your practice. It gives you not only a chance to rest and recuperate, but also the time to observe the effect of the previous asanas.

The number of times you need to include Savasana in your practice will vary from person to person, but generally it should follow standing poses and should be held for an interval of one to three minutes. You can also include it after inverted postures such as Sirsasana *(Fig. 2.35)*, Sarvangasana *(Fig. 2.36)* and Halasana *(Fig. 2.22)* and you can use it again at the end of the practice for five to ten minutes before Pranayama.

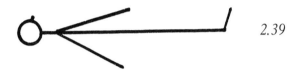

2.39

Questions

1 Which counter-posture would you give to the asanas in Fig. 2.40, and why?

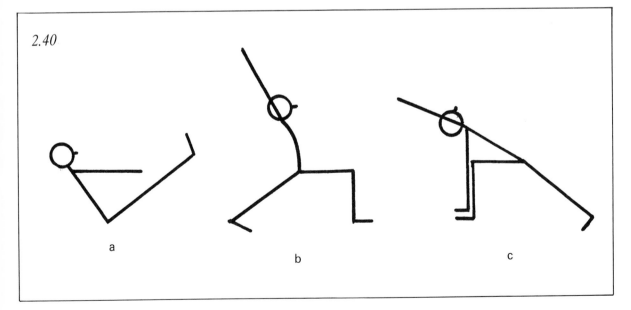

2.40

a

b

c

2 Fill in the counter-poses in the sequence in Fig. 2.41

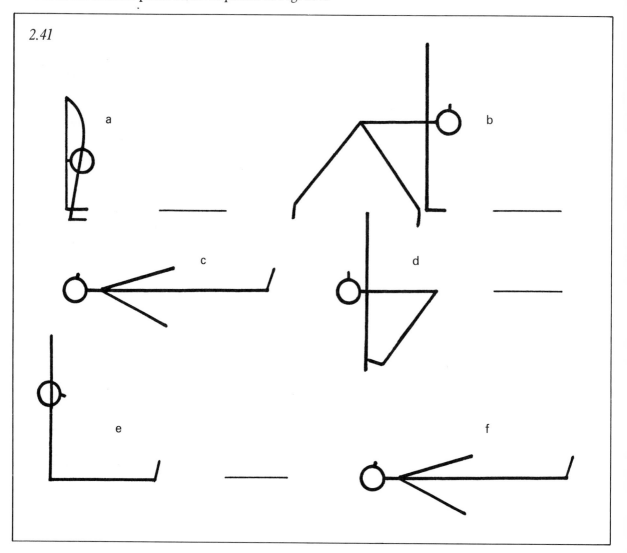

2.41

CHAPTER 3

Use of the Breath in Asanas

This chapter outlines the main principles of the precise use of breath during the practice of asanas. However, it must be stressed from the outset that the personal guidance of a suitably qualified teacher is absolutely essential.

According to the philosophy of yoga, there is a fundamental relationship between the mind and the breath. In the first chapter of Patanjali's Sutras, irregular breath is described as one of the symptoms of an unsteady wind. When we are angry, frightened or disturbed, the quality of the breath becomes shorter, faster and irregular *(Fig. 3.1a)*. Similarly, when we are relaxed and calm the quality of the breath is regular, smooth and even *(Fig. 3.1b and c)*.

Yoga has, for thousands of years, recognised the importance of this relationship between mind and breath, and uses it to help develop the mind towards a heightened perception. While Pranayama is the principal discipline in this direction, the practice of asanas, particularly when the breath is used very precisely, is an important preparation which links and integrates asanas and Pranayama.

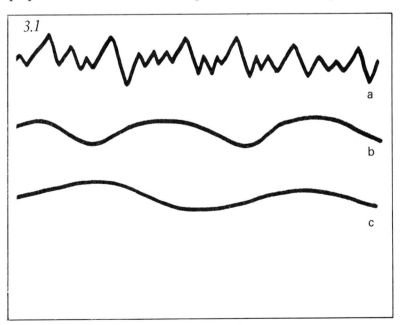

3.1

Principles of breathing in asanas

The aim of breathing in asanas is to maintain a harmony between the movement of the body and the movement of the breath. Expanding movements are therefore usually made on inhalation so that, when the body is making an opening movement, the chest and abdomen are also expanding *(Fig. 3.2)*.

Similarly, contracting movements are usually made on exhalation, when the chest and abdomen are also contracting *(Fig. 3.3)*. Twisting movements *(Fig. 3.4)* are also usually made on exhalation, as the restricting movement of the body helps to empty the lungs. Further examples are given in Fig. 3.5a-d.

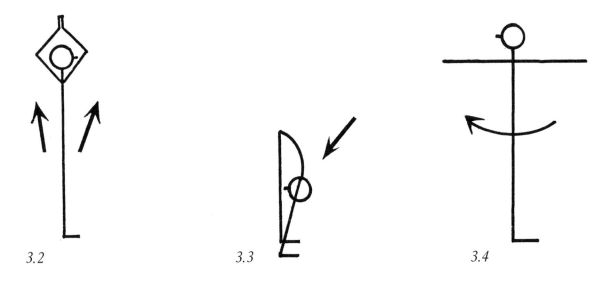

3.2   3.3   3.4

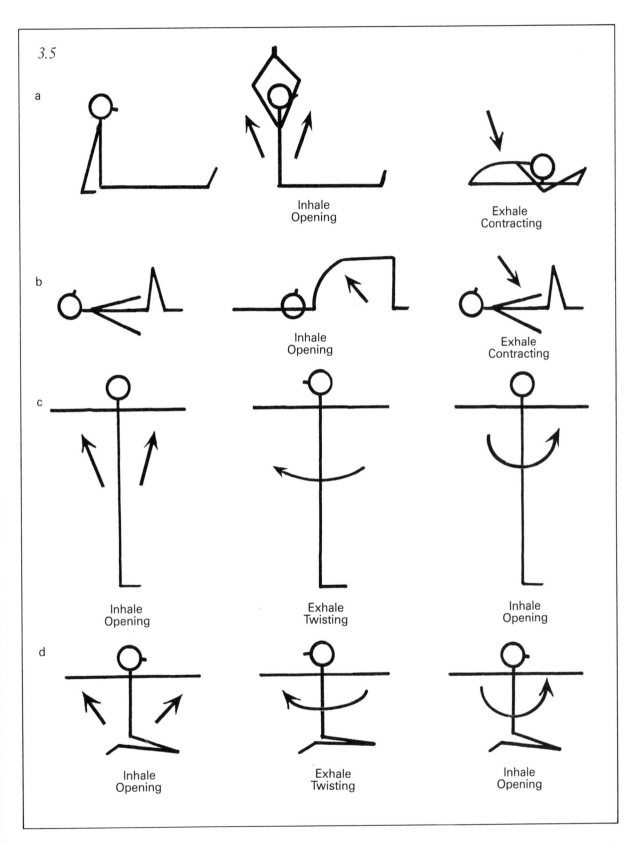

3.5

a

Inhale
Opening

Exhale
Contracting

b

Inhale
Opening

Exhale
Contracting

c

Inhale
Opening

Exhale
Twisting

Inhale
Opening

d

Inhale
Opening

Exhale
Twisting

Inhale
Opening

Leg-raising movements are usually made on exhalation because the movement of the legs has a contracting effect on the abdomen *(Fig. 3.6)*. If this movement were to be made on an inhalation, there would be a conflict between the movement of the legs, compressing the abdomen, and the movement of the lungs, which would be moving down into the abdomen as they expanded.

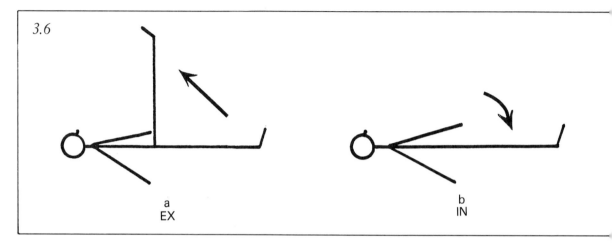

3.6

a
EX

b
IN

Synchronisation of breath and movement

Synchronisation of breath and movement adds a very important dimension to your practice and encourages concentration — it is impossible to work precisely with the breath unless the mind is concentrated and present in the practice.

Each breath should start just before the movement begins and should continue until just after the movement has finished *(Fig. 3.7)*. In this way each breath determines the speed of the movement. If your breath finishes before the movement, either the breath should be lengthened or you should increase the speed of the movement so that you complete it before the end of that breath.

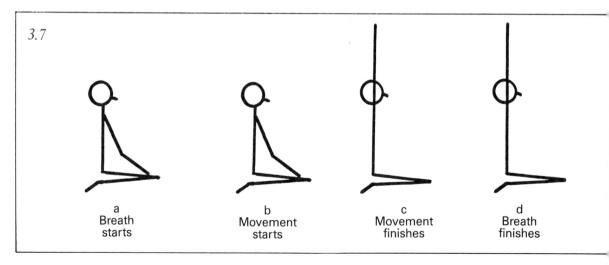

3.7

a
Breath
starts

b
Movement
starts

c
Movement
finishes

d
Breath
finishes

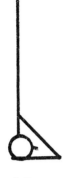

Quality of the breath

The quality of the breath has a profound effect upon each movement and posture and upon the whole of the practice itself. It should be even and refined during each inhalation and exhalation throughout your practice.

Different methods of breathing in postures

Several different types of breathing are used in the practice of asanas.

You can use nostril breathing in two ways — consciously and unconsciously. When you are first learning the postures and are having to concentrate more on the movement, it should be unconscious, as in normal breathing. As you become more familiar with the postures, you can practise nostril breathing consciously, with your attention focused on the sound, length and quality of your breath.

Throat breathing controls the breath at the throat by slightly constricting the glottis. In this way the breath can be slightly restricted, resulting in a sound which should be only just audible and soft in quality, not harsh and loud.

In some postures, such as Sirsasana *(Fig. 3.8)* Sitali breathing can be practised. This involves sucking in air through the tongue *(Fig. 3.9)* on inhalation and exhaling through the nostrils (see also Chapter 9).

3.8

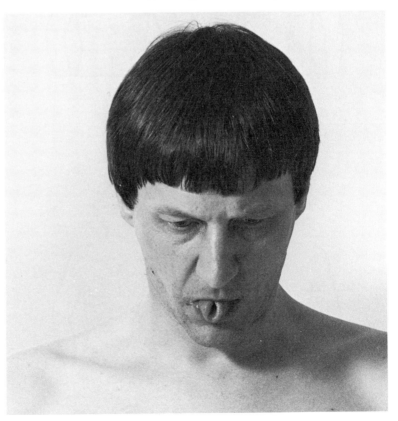

3.9

Chest movement

There are two distinctly different ways to fill the lungs. The first is to begin by filling the bottom of the lungs and then to work up to the top *(Fig. 3.10)*. The second is to fill the top of the lungs first and then work down *(Fig. 3.11)*. (For a fuller explanation see Chapter 9 on Pranayama.)

The first method of filling the lungs, from the bottom, is the best method for beginners and students who are tense. When you have achieved more control of the breath through practice, you can introduce the second, slightly more subtle, method of breathing. In this latter way, by filling the upper chest first and working downwards towards the abdomen, you can produce more movement in the upper chest. Exhalation begins from the bottom of the lungs and works upwards.

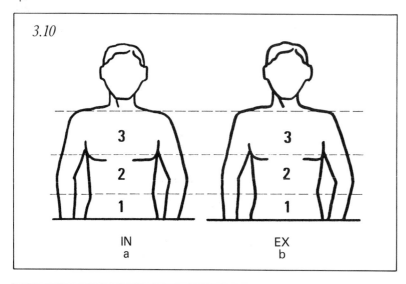

3.10

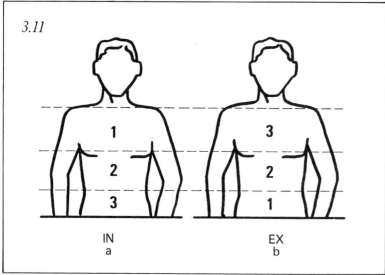

3.11

Factors which influence the breath are as follows:

1 Concentration — when you are not concentrating on the breath, the effect of the breath will be less.
2 Physical condition — when your general fitness is low your breath will tend to be short and difficult to sustain for any length of time.
3 Breathing capacity — restricted breathing capacity will shorten your breath. Good expansion and contraction of the chest and diaphragm and good control of chest movement will produce much better breathing.
4 Type of asana — postures which are very demanding will tend to make your breath shorter than ones which are less strenuous.

The following examples show how the length of the breath may be influenced by the posture. In Savasana *(Fig. 3.12)* there is no demand on your body and the breath will be longer. In Virabhadrasana *(Fig. 3.13)*, however — a much more strenuous posture — your breath will be shorter. With Sarvangasana *(Fig. 3.14)* you will find it harder to extend the inhalation because your upper chest is restricted and the diaphragm has the weight of your legs and lower body to push against. In Bhujangasana *(Fig. 3.15)* your abdomen is pressed against the ground and cannot move outward and this will often shorten the breath.

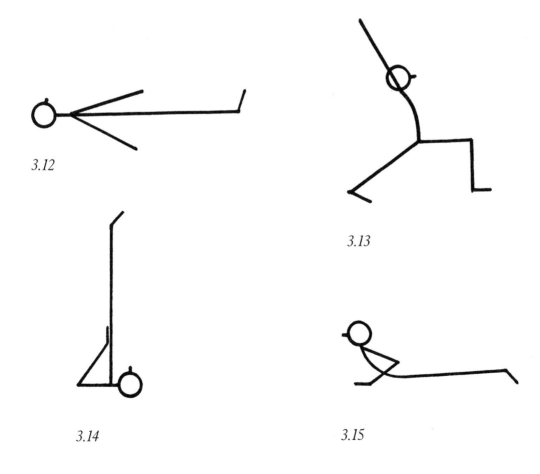

3.12

3.13

3.14

3.15

Dynamic and static use of postures

Working dynamically or statically in a posture will produce different effects upon the breath. Some postures are easier when used dynamically and some are harder. The same is true of postures used statically. In either case, the more demanding the posture the more difficult it will be for you to control your breath.

Breathing ratios

The synchronisation of breath and posture will bring a great deal of refinement into your practice. You can develop this further by using particular breathing 'ratios' with the asanas. These ratios are described in more detail in the chapter on Pranayama (Chapter 9). As an example, though, a ratio of 1:2 would mean that you make the exhalation twice as long as the inhalation:
IN (6 seconds) : EX (12 seconds)
or:
IN (10 seconds) : EX (20 seconds)
(Measuring the length of the breath can be done by mentally counting or by using a metronome set at one beat a second.)

In addition, the numbers used in breathing ratio instructions in yoga can indicate not only inhalation and exhalation but also whether the breath is held for a time after inhalation or exhalation. Thus a ratio written as 1:1:2:1 would instruct you to inhale for, let us say, six seconds, hold the breath for six seconds, exhale for twelve seconds and again hold the breath for six seconds:
IN (6) : H (6) : EX (12) : H (6)
The six seconds is a random choice; using the same ratio you could inhale for ten seconds, hold for ten, exhale for twenty and hold again for ten, or choose any comfortable length of time, so long as the ratio remains the same:
IN (10) : H (10) : EX (20) : H (10)
or:
IN (8) : H (8) : EX (16) : H (8)
Where there is no retention of the breath after the inhalation or exhalation, a zero is often used, e.g.:
IN (5) : H (0) : EX (10) : H (0)
Retention only after inhalation would thus be:
5 : 5 : 10 : 0
and retention only after exhalation would be:
5 : 0 : 10 : 5
Normally we breathe to a 1:1½ ratio, with the exhalation half as long again as the inhalation, e.g.
IN (4) : EX (6)
When using ratios in yoga this natural breathing ratio is consciously developed to achieve a greater control of the breath.

It should be stressed that retention of the breath in postures needs to be practised with proper supervision.

Types of ratio

Ratios without retention
Since the normal breathing ratio is $1:1\frac{1}{2}$, the easiest ratios to use are $1:1, 1:1\frac{1}{4}, 1:1\frac{1}{2}$ and $1:2$ (see Figs 3.16, 3.17, 3.18 and 3.18a).

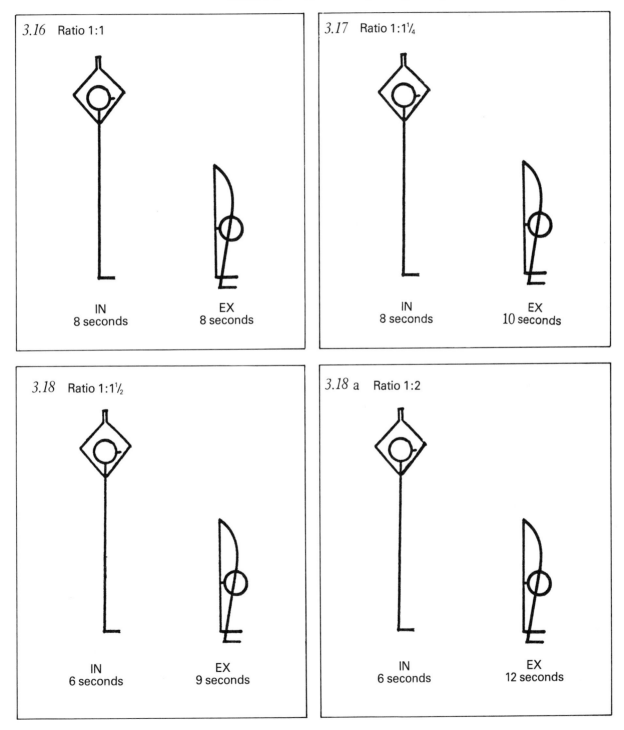

3.16 Ratio 1:1

IN
8 seconds

EX
8 seconds

3.17 Ratio $1:1\frac{1}{4}$

IN
8 seconds

EX
10 seconds

3.18 Ratio $1:1\frac{1}{2}$

IN
6 seconds

EX
9 seconds

3.18 a Ratio 1:2

IN
6 seconds

EX
12 seconds

Ratios with retention

Retention of the breath will greatly intensify the effect of an asana, but you should only practise it with the direct guidance of a teacher. Such breath retention falls into two categories:

1 ratios with retention after inhalation (see Fig. 3.19);
2 ratios with retention after exhalation (see Fig. 3.20).

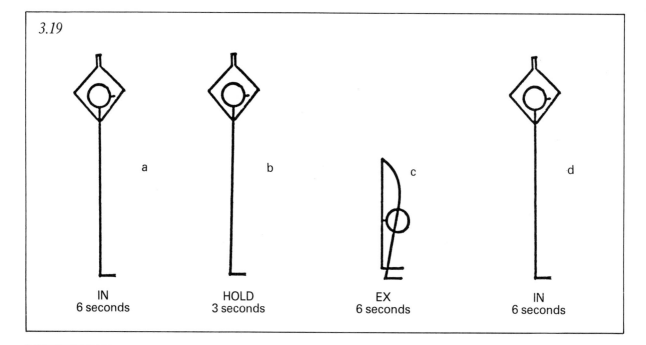

3.19

a	b	c	d
IN	HOLD	EX	IN
6 seconds	3 seconds	6 seconds	6 seconds

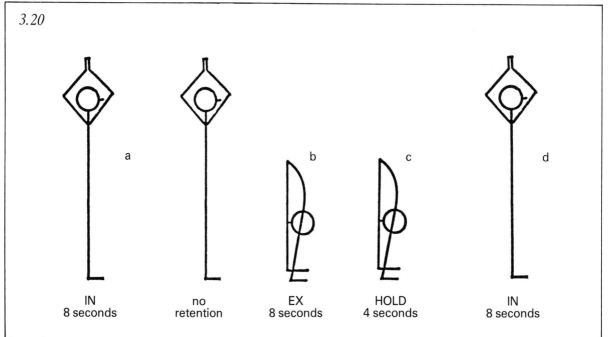

3.20

a	b	c	d
IN	no	EX	HOLD	IN
8 seconds	retention	8 seconds	4 seconds	8 seconds

As has already been said, different asanas affect the breath in different ways. Some postures are more suitable for holding after inhalation, some after exhalation and some after both.

1 Fig. 3.21 shows some examples of postures more suitable for retaining the breath after inhalation.
2 The postures in Fig. 3.22 are more suitable for retaining the breath after exhalation.

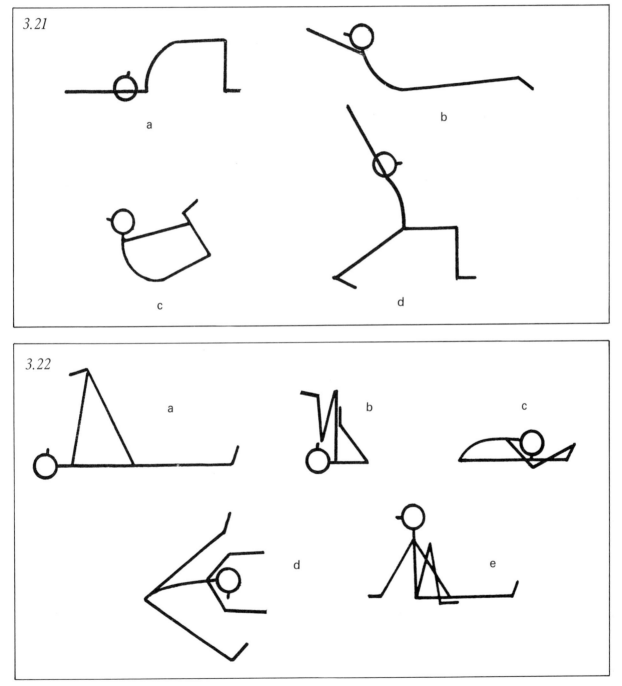

3 The postures in Fig. 3.23 are suitable for retention of the breath after inhalation and exhalation.

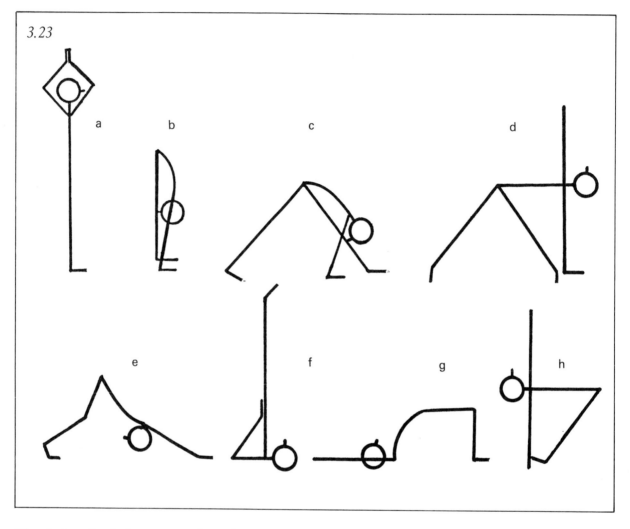

3.23

The choice of ratio for an asana depends, to some extent, on whether you are using the posture dynamically or statically. For example, Pascimatanasana *(Fig. 3.24)*, if held statically, is usually more effective if the breath is held after exhalation. However, if you use it dynamically, so that your body comes up from the posture on inhalation, then retention of the breath could follow inhalation *(Fig. 3.25)*.

Additionally, you can use Pascimatanasana dynamically with retention of the breath after inhalation and exhalation *(Fig. 3.26)*. This breathing ratio could also be used in the same way in Vajrasana *(Fig. 3.27)*.

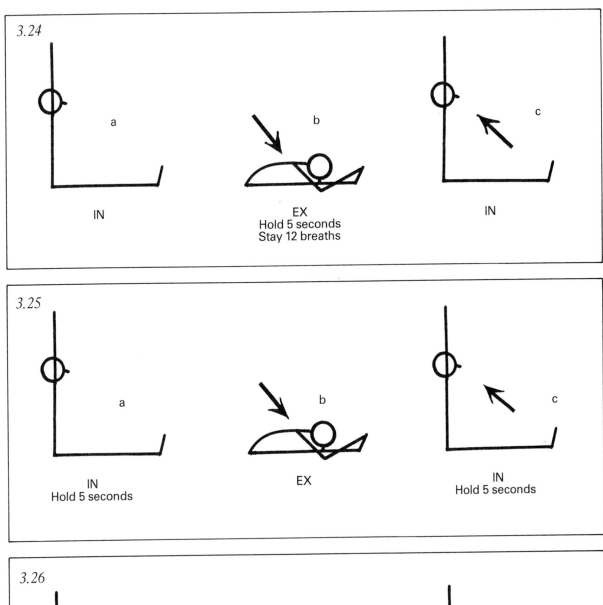

3.24

a — IN

b — EX
Hold 5 seconds
Stay 12 breaths

c — IN

3.25

a — IN
Hold 5 seconds

b — EX

c — IN
Hold 5 seconds

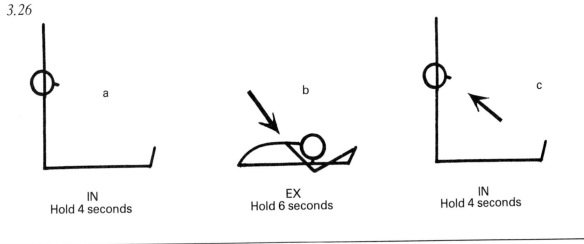

3.26

a — IN
Hold 4 seconds

b — EX
Hold 6 seconds

c — IN
Hold 4 seconds

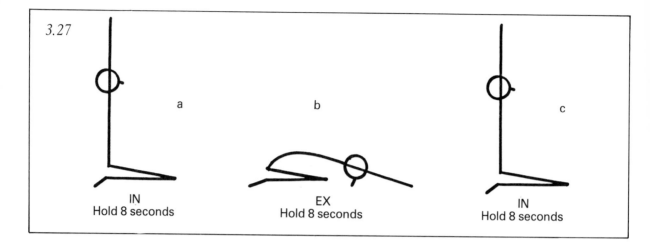

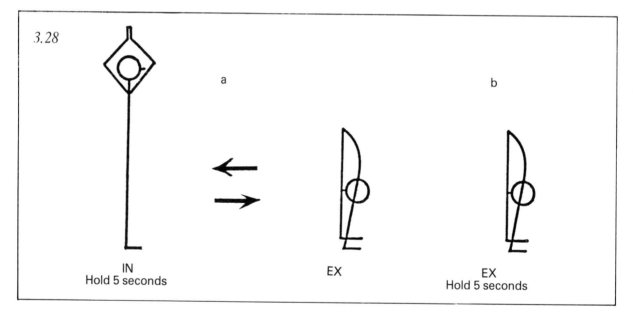

Combining different ratios

It is often useful to combine different types of ratios within one posture. For example Uttanasana can be used dynamically with retention after inhalation and then used statically with retention after exhalation *(Fig. 3.28)*. Retention in each case will accentuate the effect of the dynamic or static use of the asana.

Choice of ratio

Normally retention of the breath in postures should not be longer than the length of the inhalation. You should exercise particular caution when retaining the breath in inverted postures and, again, you should only attempt this under the guidance of your teacher.

Mental and physical condition are factors which influence the choice of ratios.

Mental condition

If you are tense it is generally better to practise without retention of the breath. A longer exhalation is usually more relaxing. Sometimes a short retention of two or three seconds after either inhalation or exhalation may be helpful.

If you are feeling lethargic it is often useful to introduce retention after inhalation, providing of course there are no other factors which need to be considered, such as high blood-pressure.

When you are feeling mentally relaxed and balanced you can practise retention after inhalation and exhalation, providing you take your physical condition into account.

Physical condition

There are so many variable factors concerning physical condition that it is really impossible to give general guidelines. You will need the advice of your teacher.

Advantages of working with the breath in asana

You can increase your breathing capacity more effectively by consciously working with the breath throughout the practice than would otherwise be possible with unconscious breathing.

The breath also acts as a gauge in measuring the effects of the asanas. When it becomes shorter and harder to control, it indicates immediately that the postures are becoming a strain.

You can measure the amount of time you have spent in each posture by counting the number of breaths. For example, staying in Pascimatanasana with a breathing ratio of 10:0:20:0 seconds for twenty breaths will take five minutes. You will find this method of measuring the time spent in practice quite useful when attempting gradually to increase the time a posture is held. If your aim is, say, to hold Sarvangasana for six minutes, it would be possible to practise holding it in the following progressions:

> 1st month 5:0:10:0 × 12 breaths = 3 minutes
> 2nd month 5:0:10:0 × 18 breaths = $4\frac{1}{2}$ minutes
> 3rd month 5:0:10:0 × 24 breaths = 6 minutes

Working with the breath helps with observation of inherent breathing problems and makes it possible to choose a ratio which will be particularly useful in reducing these problems. For example, you may have difficulty in controlling exhalation, both in Pranayama and asanas. By giving a longer exhalation in suitable asanas you will probably overcome this weakness.

Conscious breathing in asanas, particularly when practised with retention, helps to unify the practice of asanas and Pranayama. Preparing both physically and mentally for a particular ratio in Pranayama by using the same ratio, or one similar to it, in your practice of asanas will improve the quality of Pranayama.

Questions and observations

1 Observe your own practice and note the breathing ratio you use naturally in different postures.
2 What breathing ratios would be suitable in the asanas in Fig. 3.29?

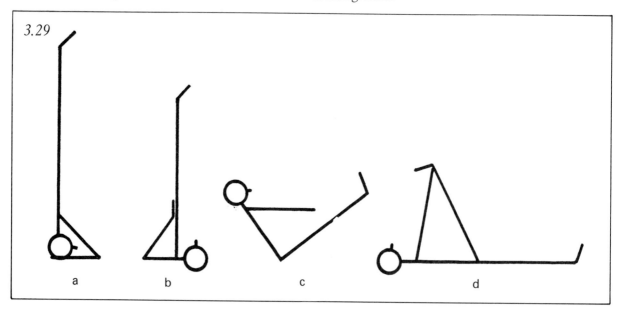

3.29

a   b   c   d

3 Compare the effects of the postures and ratios in Fig. 3.30 and 3.31.

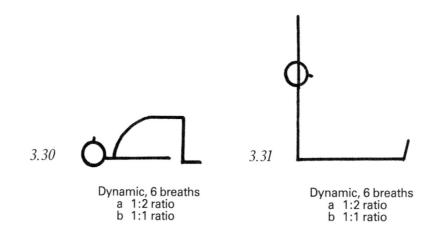

3.30

Dynamic, 6 breaths
a 1:2 ratio
b 1:1 ratio

3.31

Dynamic, 6 breaths
a 1:2 ratio
b 1:1 ratio

CHAPTER 4

Asanas Used Statically and Dynamically

The static and dynamic use of asanas will add another important dimension to your practice. It allows you to develop a great deal of variety in the way you can use each posture and, as a result, you can direct your practice more effectively to your own needs.

There are three possible ways in which to move in asanas.

1 Statically — to move into a posture and stay in that position.
2 Dynamically — to repeat the movement several times.
3 A combination of both.

Asanas used dynamically

When you are working dynamically in a posture you repeat the whole movement in order to work particular parts of the body *(Fig. 4.1)*.

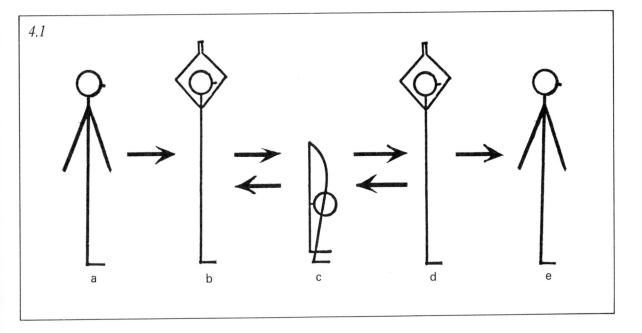

4.1

a   b   c   d   e

Some postures are physically more strenuous when used dynamically, although to some extent this will vary from person to person. For example, if you are stiff but strong you will find it easier to work dynamically in Parsva Uttanasana *(Fig. 4.2),* while if you are weak but supple you will find it easier to work statically.

The postures in Fig. 4.3 are generally easier when used dynamically, while those in Fig. 4.4 are generally more strenuous.

4.2

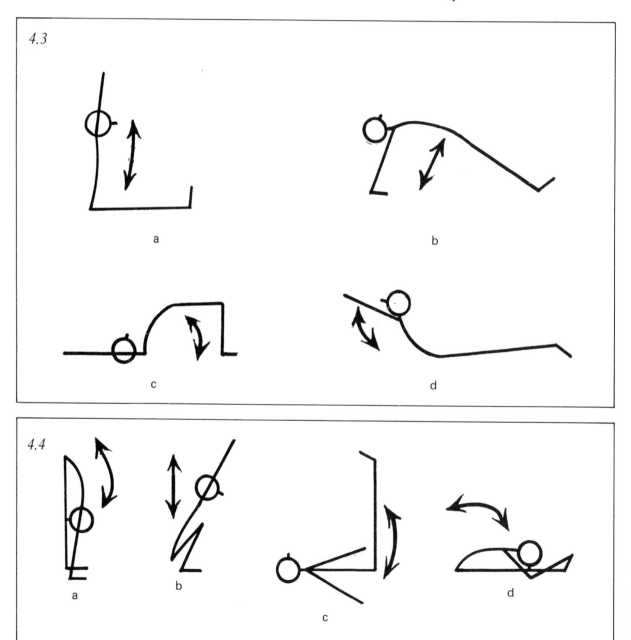

4.3

a

b

c

d

4.4

a

b

c

d

Dynamic movements

There are many ways of working dynamically in postures. The following will give you some idea of the possibilities.

Uttanasana

1 Uninterrupted movement into the complete position and back again *(Fig. 4.5)*.

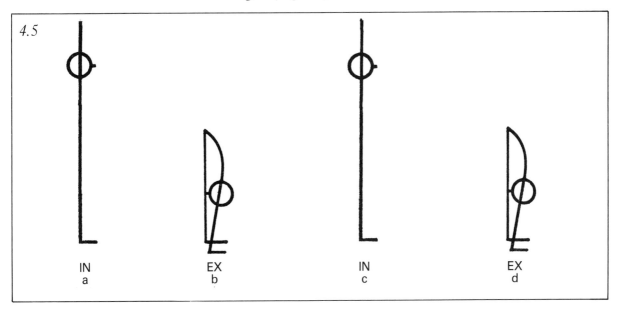

4.5

IN   EX   IN   EX
a   b   c   d

2 Stopping the movement when coming up from the posture *(Fig. 4.6)*.

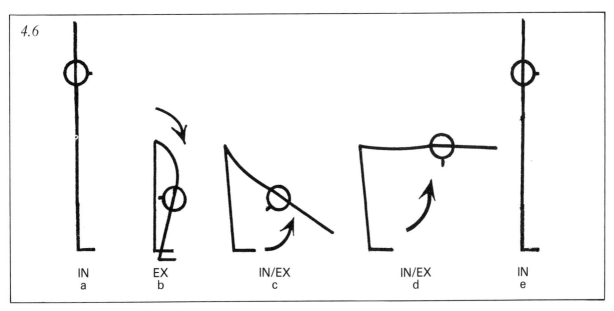

4.6

IN   EX   IN/EX   IN/EX   IN
a   b   c   d   e

3 Stopping the movement when going down into the posture (*Fig. 4.7*).

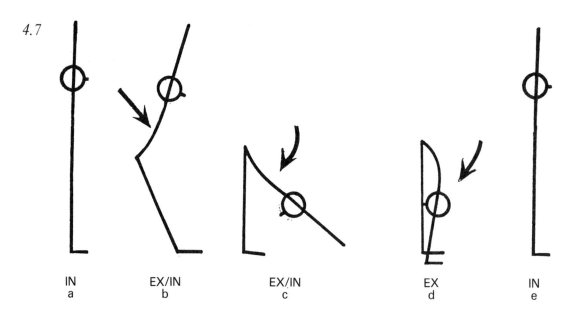

4.7

IN	EX/IN	EX/IN	EX	IN
a	b	c	d	e

4 Combinations of stopping the movement when going down into the posture and when coming up. In Fig. 4.8 the movement is downward on an exhalation and is held half-way.

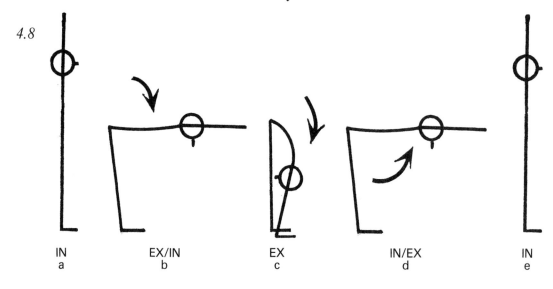

4.8

IN	EX/IN	EX	IN/EX	IN
a	b	c	d	e

Advantages of working dynamically

Dynamic movement adds a great deal of mental and physical refinement; with even a very simple posture such as Uttanasana an enormous number of movements are possible.

Physiological advantages

1 Working dynamically is the best way of warming up your body. Standing postures in particular, if used dynamically at the beginning of your practice, will be very effective in preparing the whole body for other asanas.

2 By repeating a movement you will find it easier to assess the quality of the breath. The breath rarely remains the same from day to day and you therefore need to see each day how it is responding in postures. Because working dynamically is often physically more demanding than remaining statically in a posture, the quality of the breath quickly becomes apparent.

3 If you want to work in a posture which is difficult to hold statically you could begin by working in it dynamically. This will gradually strengthen those parts of the body used most, and will also prepare the breath. For example if your aim is to hold Bhujangasana *(Fig. 4.9)* statically for twelve breaths, you could begin by working dynamically, gradually increasing the time spent in the posture until you are sufficiently prepared to work statically.

4 When the dynamic use of postures intensifies the effect of an asana it becomes more effective in strengthening weak areas of the body. For example, Uttanasana *(Fig. 4.5)* could be beneficial in helping strengthen a weak back (provided the back is not *too* weak, in which case it may cause pain).

5 Working dynamically also helps increase flexibility. If you are stiff and the forward movement in Pascimatanasana *(Fig. 4.10)* is restricted, then working dynamically will be the most effective way for you to loosen the stiff area.

6 Working dynamically is also useful in counter-poses that help remove the negative effects of a posture. For example, if you have held Uttanasana statically for twelve breaths, you can use Utkatasana *(Fig. 4.11)* dynamically.

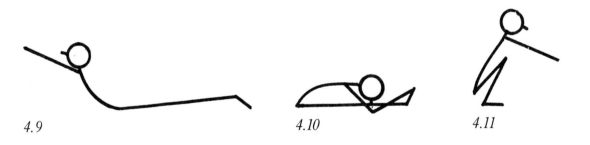

4.9 *4.10* *4.11*

Psychological advantages

With dynamic movements an enormous number of different permutations become possible and these should help you vary your practice and maintain interest and concentration.

Asanas used statically

Working statically in a posture, after adequate preparation, is usually more beneficial if your body is supple and strong enough to move all the way into the asana and can then remain there comfortably. (However, if you are stiff or if your back is supple but weak, and needs strengthening, a dynamic movement is usually better.)

Physiological advantages

1 By staying in a forward-bending posture you can stretch completely into a pose.
2 When asanas are intensified by holding, the body is strengthened, stretched or bent more effectively, as in Fig. 4.12.
3 Using very easy postures statically, especially in counter-poses, gives the body a chance to rest and recover, as in Fig. 4.13.
4 You can pay more attention to the breath when a posture is held statically, and the mind can become more absorbed in this aspect of the practice. Retention of the breath is also easier because there is less exertion.

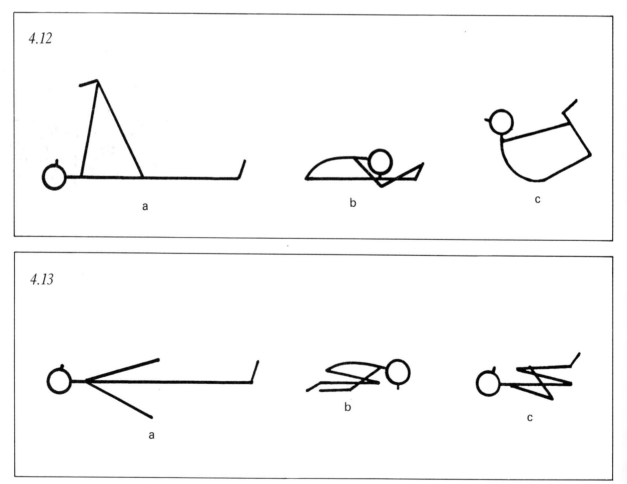

4.12
a b c

4.13
a b c

Psychological advantages

When a posture is held, the psychological effects are more pronounced than when dynamic movements are used. Postures which have a physically opening effect have a similar mental effect; conversely, contracting postures tend to have an introverting mental effect. For example, the psychological effects of staying in Pascimatanasana for twenty breaths will be very different to those produced by working dynamically in the pose for twenty breaths.

Asanas used statically and dynamically

Working dynamically and statically can produce a number of new permutations *(Fig. 4.14)*. In this Figure the dynamic movements help prepare for the posture to be held statically.

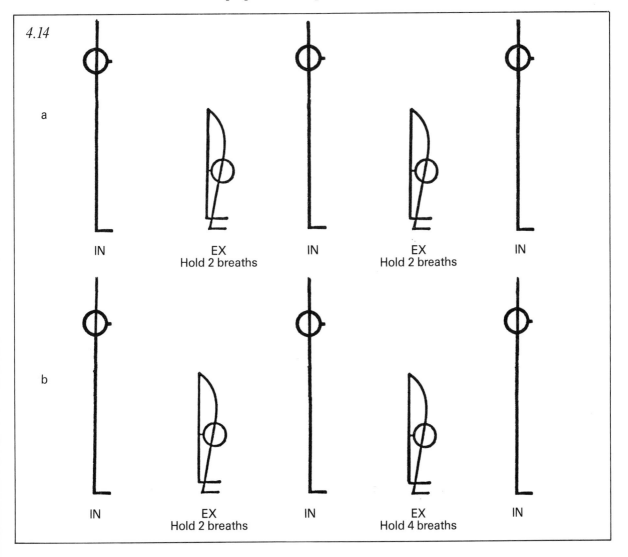

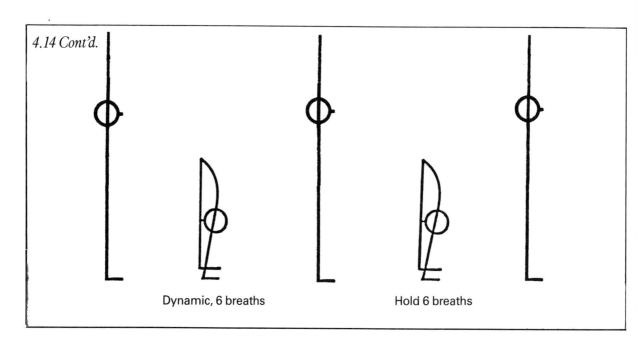

4.14 Cont'd.

Dynamic, 6 breaths   Hold 6 breaths

Questions and observations

1 Compare Dvipada Pitham *(Fig. 4.15)* held for:
   a eight breaths statically;
   b eight breaths dynamically;
   NB Use the same breathing ratio.

4.15

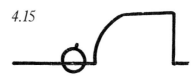

2 How many ways of working dynamically are there in the asanas in
   Fig. 4.16?

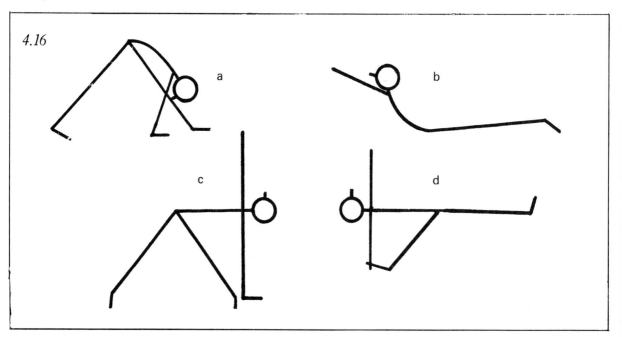

4.16

3 Taking the sequence of postures in Fig. 4.17, compare its use when practised:
a dynamically;
b statically;
with six breaths for each pose.

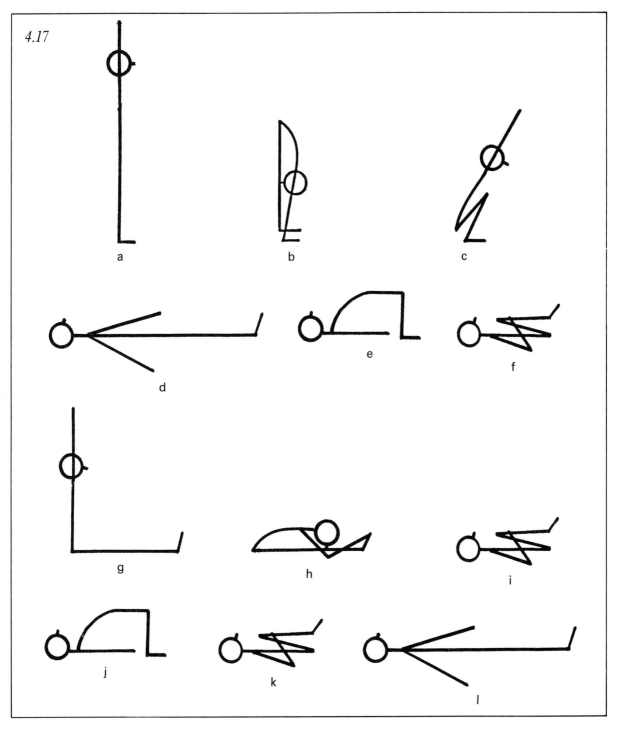

4.17

a

b

c

d

e

f

g

h

i

j

k

l

CHAPTER 5

Variations of Asanas

Many of the classical asanas of Yoga are well known; Sarvangasana *(Fig. 5.1)*, Pascimatanasana *(Fig. 5.2)*, Padmasana *(Fig. 5.3)* and Adhomukha Svanasana *(Fig. 5.4)* are postures usually included in books on Yoga and are taught in many Yoga classes. What may not be so well-known is that most asanas have a large number of variations, the use of which makes the practice of asanas more effective, both physically and mentally.

5.1

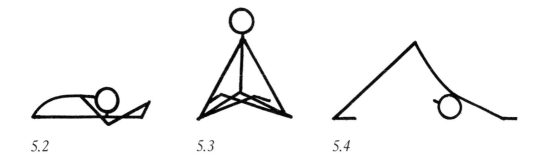

5.2   *5.3*   *5.4*

Variations are used in a number of ways to make postures easier or harder, and they can also be used to develop balance and to loosen particular joints or muscles. Additionally, different variations can develop a particular aspect of breathing in a posture. Variations change classical postures by combining them with classical movements and positions of the arms and legs and thus altering the effects of the postures.

If, for example, you have stiff shoulders, it is possible to use particular variations of postures which will work the shoulders far more than the classical asanas. For example, you could use Parsva Uttanasana *(Fig. 5.5)* and Vajrasana *(Fig. 5.6)* with the arms swept behind the back. Other postures you could use with movement of the arms include Tadasana *(Fig. 5.7)*, Pascimatanasana *(Fig. 5.8)* and Bhujangasana *(Fig. 5.9)*. In all the postures in Fig. 5.7—5.9 there is a movement of the arms.

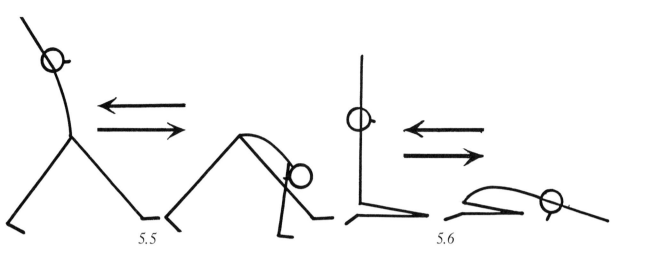

5.5

5.6

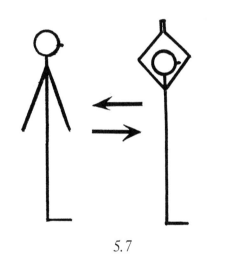

5.7

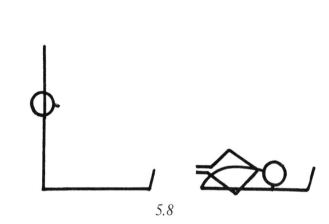

5.8

5.9

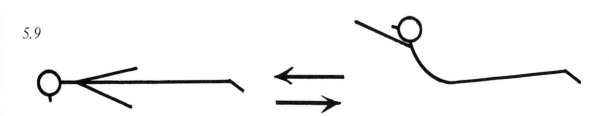

Similarly, in Uttanasana *(Fig. 5.10)* the arms could be swept behind the back as the body moves down into the posture and then brought back as the body comes up from the pose.

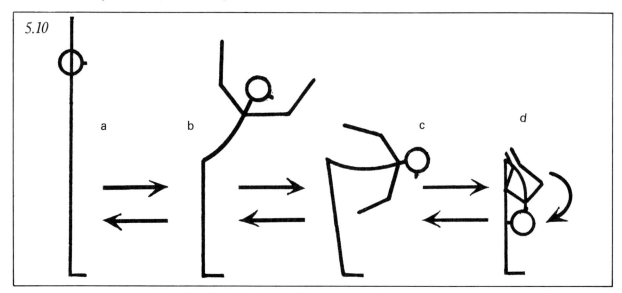

Another example where variations are useful would be if your back was weaker on one side. Here, asymmetrical variations could isolate the weak side of your back and ensure that it was worked and strengthened *(Fig. 5.11)*.

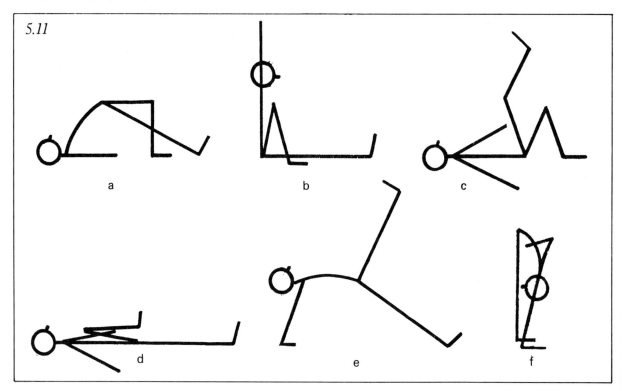

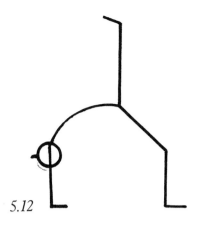

5.12

Variations and Vinyasa

The use of variations also plays an important part in preparing areas of the body for a particular main posture, or a posture in a Vinyasa which may itself be a variation of a classical asana. For example, if Ekapada Urdhva Dhanurasana *(Fig. 5.12)* was to be the main posture in your practice, the variations in Fig. 5.13 might be useful preparations. It should be stressed, however, that asymmetrical postures should be practised on *both* sides.

Padmasana *(Fig. 5.14)* is another example of a classical asana for which you can use variations as preparation. Variations in standing, inverted and lying postures could be used, as in Fig. 5.15.

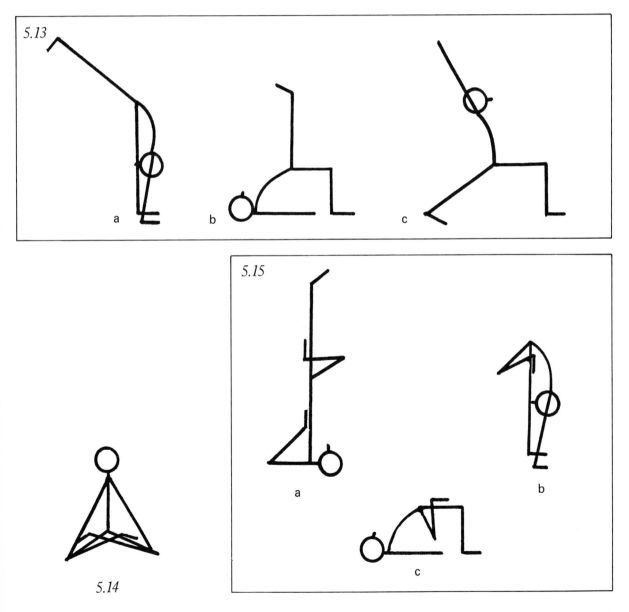

5.13
a b c

5.15
a b c

5.14

Benefit of variations

There are a number of mental benefits to be gained from using variations. There is always a danger when we do something regularly that it may become a dull routine and that our minds will not be fully attentive. If this happens to you, then one of the main aims of your practice has been lost. By introducing different variations of the classical postures you will experience the asanas in a different way and this will develop a more creative and imaginative approach.

You can also use variations to develop a deeper concentration during your practice. If an asana is used dynamically, there is always the tendency for it to become automatic after the first few movements. With the introduction of one or more variations you can overcome or greatly reduce this tendency. Dvipada Pitham *(Fig. 5.16)* and its variations *(Fig. 5.17)* are a good illustration. You could use several variations of the same posture within one practice or separately over a number of days.

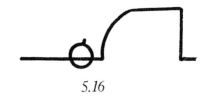

5.16

Another important use of variations comes into play in the relationship between the teacher and the pupil. One of the most important features of teaching is the relationship and level of communication between teacher and pupil. If the teacher, by careful observation, can give a student personal variations it demonstrates, on the one hand, his awareness of the student's individual needs while, on the other hand, it helps the pupil to feel the sincere interest of the teacher.

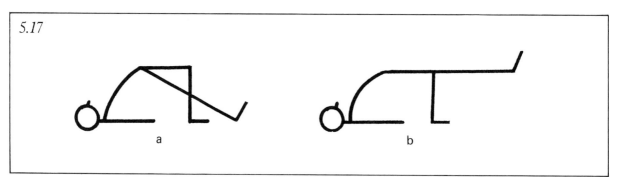

5.17

a

b

Variations of Uttanasana

To help illustrate the number of variations and their uses more fully it might be useful to take one posture such as Uttanasana *(Fig. 5.18)* and analyse it in detail. You should remember that the effects of a posture will vary a great deal from person to person, so the notes are of a very general nature.

Uttanasana stretches the back and the backs of the legs, and works the shoulders and arms. Sweeping the arms behind the back works the shoulders and makes the posture less demanding on the back *(Fig. 5.19)*. This variation would be useful if you had stiff shoulders and/or a problem in your back which would make working with the arms straight out in front too difficult.

5.18

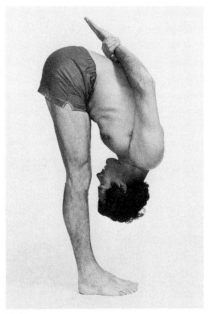

5.19

A variation of this kind is also useful when working with a particular breathing ratio. For example, if there is retention of the breath after inhalation, a less strenuous variation would be more appropriate in some cases in order to make the retention of the breath easier.

The arms can be placed behind the back in a number of positions. A simple variation is with the hands resting on the lower back and the fingers interlocked *(Fig. 5.20)* or with the hands holding the elbows *(Fig. 5.21)*. Another variation is with the palms together and the fingers pointing down *(Fig. 5.22)*, while a harder variation is with the palms together and the fingers facing up *(Fig. 5.23)* — this works the wrist more than with the fingers pointing down. All these variations can be useful if you have a tendency to round your shoulders while moving into the posture; when your arms are behind your back your chest is kept open and your shoulders are kept back.

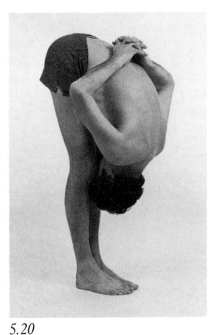

5.20

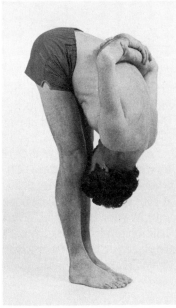

5.21

5.22

Other variations include keeping the arms behind the back with the fingers interlocked and with the arms straightened and pulled away from the body. The palms can be kept turned in *(Fig. 5.24)* or turned out *(Fig. 5.25)*. In both these variations the shoulders are flexed and the weight of the arms helps the forward-bending movement.

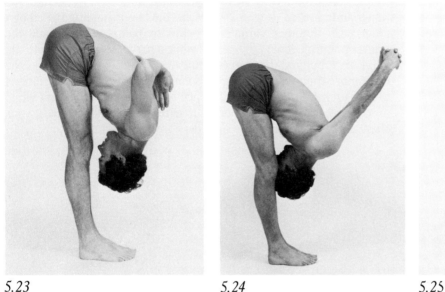

5.23   5.24   5.25

There are several variations of this posture where the arms are placed on the head. Two examples are included, one with the palms together *(Fig. 5.26)* and another with the fingers interlocked *(Fig. 5.27)*. Both of these help to keep the shoulders, neck and upper-back relaxed.

Lowering the hands to the floor *(Fig. 5.28)* gives a strong stretch to your back and helps bring your body forward into the posture. The same variation can be practised with your feet apart *(Fig. 5.29)*, making the posture easier, particularly if your sense of balance is poor.

The arms can be spread at right angles to your body *(Fig. 5.30)*, helping to keep your chest open. This variation tends to work the back more than variations where the hands are placed on the floor or where they hold your legs.

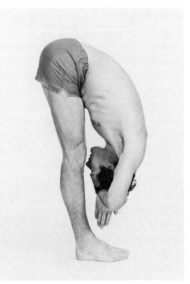

5.26

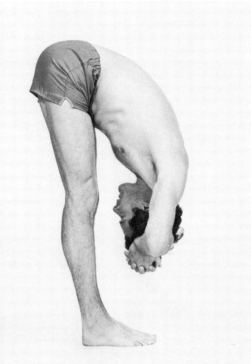

5.27

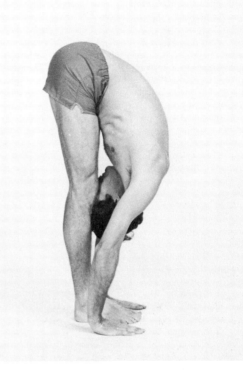

5.28

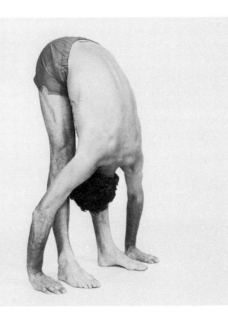

5.29

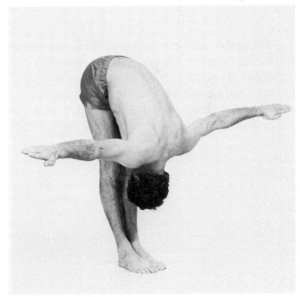

5.30

Your hands can be interlocked behind the calves of your legs, either with the palms pointing in *(Fig. 5.31)* or out *(Fig. 5.32)*. Because your hands are not placed on the floor the forward-bending movement is much harder. Another variation, where your hands are not used to help the forward-bending movement, has the hands placed on the floor facing upwards *(Fig. 5.33)*. The arms and shoulders are more relaxed and the forward stretch has to come from your lower back.

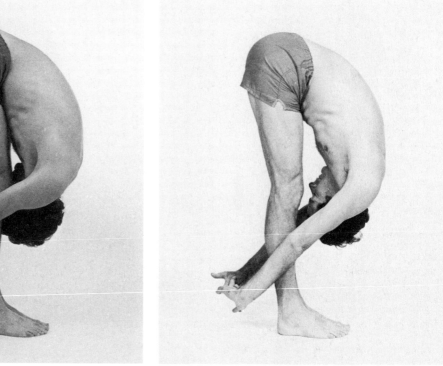

5.33

5.31   *5.32*

Holding the backs of your legs *(Fig. 5.34)*, your big toes *(Fig. 5.35)* or placing your hands under your feet *(Fig. 5.36)* are all useful variations. By pulling gently you can increase the stretch on your back and legs. You can use these variations dynamically by lifting your head and trunk on the inhalation (as shown in Figs. 5.34—5.36) and bending forward to place your head back on your knees on the exhalation.

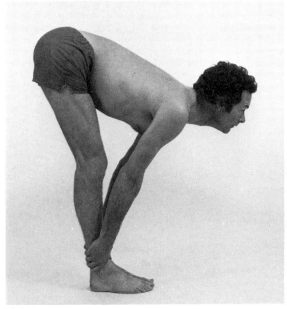

5.34

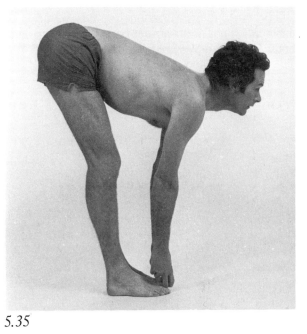

5.35

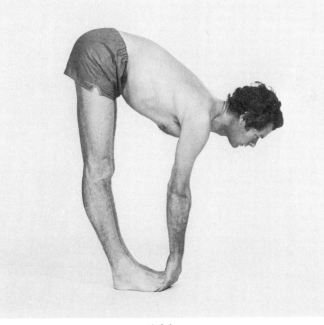

5.36

Variations on Ardha Uttanasana

Ardha Uttanasana *(Fig. 5.37)* is an excellent posture for strengthening the back. In the classical pose the arms are held in front of the head, as here, and the centre of gravity is moved towards the upper part of the back. The upper-back, lower-back and shoulders therefore have to work vigorously in order to keep the arms parallel to the floor.

There are many variations on this posture, all of which place different emphasis on various parts of the back and other parts of the body. Four examples are given in Figs. 5.38—5.41.

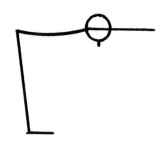

5.37

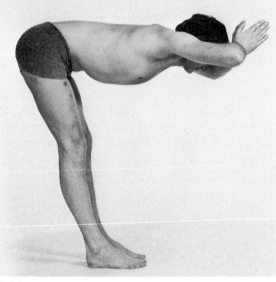

5.38

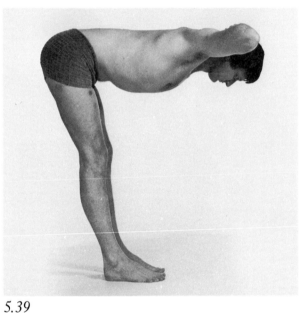

5.39

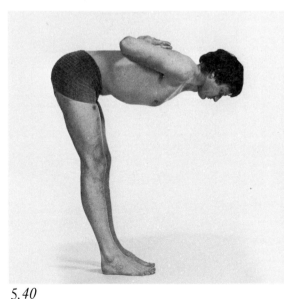

5.40

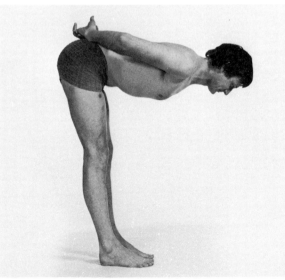

5.41

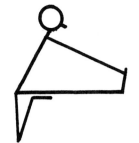

5.42

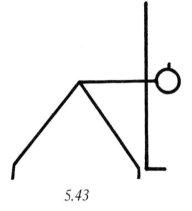

5.43

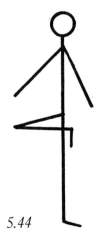

5.44

Asymmetrical variations

Asymmetrical postures play an important part in the practice of asanas. Many of the classical postures are asymmetrical, Mahamudra *(Fig. 5.42)*, Trikonasana *(Fig. 5.43)* and Bhagirathasana *(Fig. 5.44)* being examples. These postures work one side of the body more vigorously than the other.

You will probably find you have a natural preference for using one side of your body more than the other and, because it is used more, it will be stronger and more flexible. In every-day movement, and also in symmetrical postures, the stronger side of your body invariably carries the weaker side. By working with asymmetrical postures it is possible to isolate the weaker muscles or joints and ensure that they are worked effectively. Frequently these imbalances in the body are very prominent and need correcting.

Many of the classical postures have variations which are asymmetrical and you can use these in various ways depending on your individual needs. Uttanasana has a number of asymmetrical variations which will help to illustrate this point. Placing one arm behind your back is one way of making Uttanasana an asymmetrical pose *(Fig. 5.45)*. This makes one side of your back work more vigorously than the other and might be a useful variation for you if there was a marked weakness on one side.

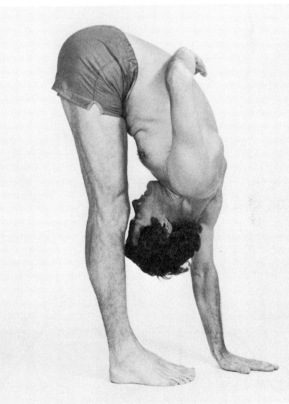

5.45

There are several other variations of Uttanasana where the body balances on one leg *(Fig. 5.46)*. These help to develop a sense of physical balance. Each leg alternately has to support the weight of the body, while one side of the back has to lift the leg up as the body moves forward. This strengthens the legs. In Fig. 5.47 one leg is held in Ardha Padmasana. This rotates the hip joint and, as one hip is thus locked, restricts the hip movement; if you are to move forward into the posture, your back therefore has to stretch more.

This examination of one posture emphasises how many ways an asana can be altered and how differrent variations will work on different parts of the body.

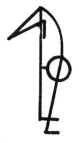

5.47

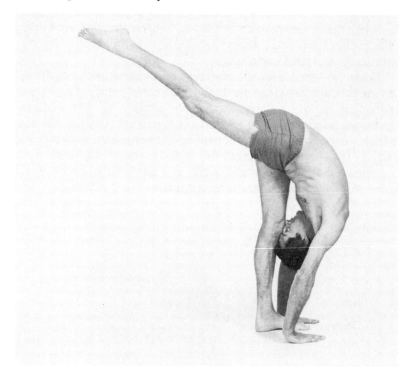

5.46

Questions and observations

1 Prepare a list of all the variations possible in the postures in Fig. 5.48.

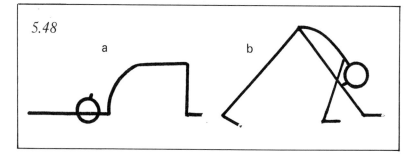

5.48
a
b

2 Compare the effects of the following variations on your lower-back, upper-back, shoulders and neck:
a see Fig. 5.49;
b see Fig. 5.50.

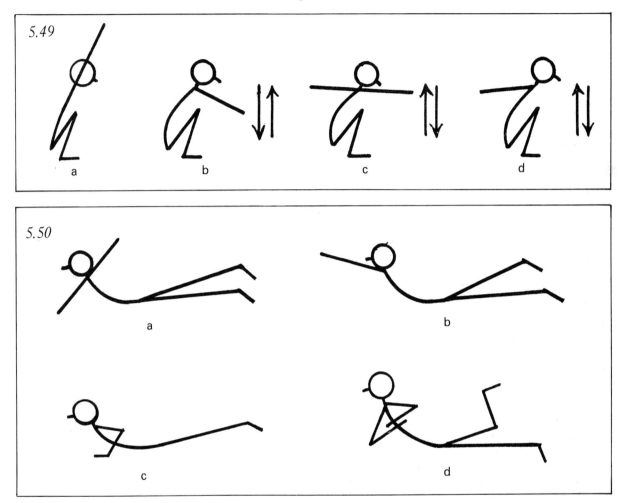

5.49

a   b   c   d

5.50

a   b

c   d

CHAPTER 6

Modifications of Asanas

In this tradition, modification plays a very important role in the practice of asanas. It can be used to make them more difficult, to work more on specific areas of the body and to add variety and interest during practice. But perhaps most important of all, at least in the West, it can make postures easier. In this way there is no need to strain oneself by trying to achieve a posture which, in the early stages, could be a physical impossibility. Instead, modifications allow you to perform asanas properly, within your own limits, and so achieve most benefit from the asana.

In the main, modifications of asanas are necessary because many people begin to practise yoga when their bodies are not in good condition. This may be due to lack of exercise, to poor diet, or to tension and stress. Whatever the reason, it often results in poor coordination, in restricted breathing and in all or particular areas of the body being stiff or weak, or both. Modifications help to avoid the danger of students in poor condition nullifying the beneficial effects of asanas by attempting too much and practising postures badly.

Asanas, modified so that they are easier, provide a way of gradually introducing postures which would otherwise be too demanding. Conversely, asanas can also be modified to make them more strenuous so that all or particular areas of the body can be worked on more effectively than in the classical postures. These two themes can best be illustrated by taking a number of postures, looking at some modifications of them, and examining the effects these modifications have.

Standing postures

Utkatasana made easier

When used dynamically, Utkatasana *(Fig. 6.1)*works quite vigorously on the thigh muscles. However, if these muscles are weak you may find the posture too demanding.

One modification to help make the posture easier is to hold on to a table-top or mantelpiece and use your arms to help pull up your body. This strengthens your arms and can also be helpful if your ankles are stiff.

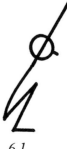

6.1

Holding on to a table-top or chair *(Fig. 6.2)* can also correct a sideways movement, which often occurs if there is stiffness in one hip or a problem in one knee or leg. With your feet on the floor and your hands anchored, it is easier to control the movement and keep your body straight. The position of the arms may also be varied *(Fig. 6.3)*, and the effects of this will differ according to the individual.

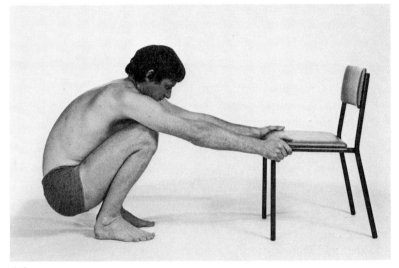

6.2

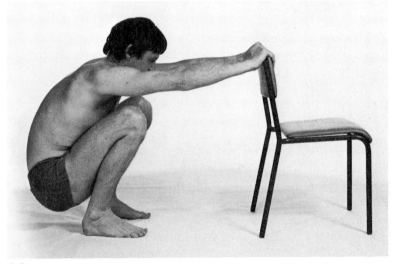

6.3

Placing a book under your heels is another modification that makes Utkatasana easier *(Fig. 6.4)*, especially if you lose your balance when you keep your heels on the floor. The book enables the heels to take the weight of your body as the ankles are flexed, which is more effective than letting your heels come up off the floor.

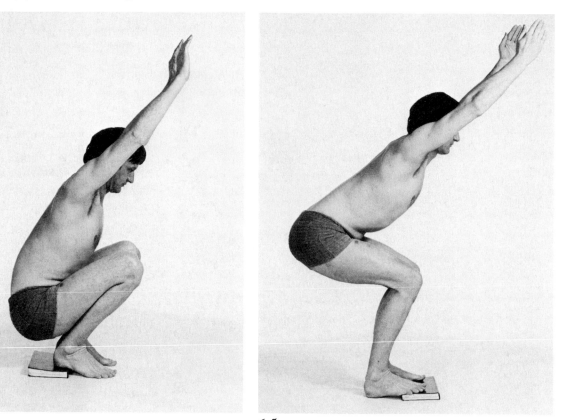

6.4

6.5

Utkatasana made harder

Placing a book under the front of your feet *(Fig. 6.5)* is a modification to make the posture much more difficult if you find the classical Utkatasana pose too easy. The effects will be especially noticeable if you have very loose hips.

By placing a book between your hands *(Fig. 6.6)* your shoulders and upper back are worked more. In this mofidication your arms can be kept above your head, they can be bent at the elbows or they can be moved up and down on the inhalation and exhalation.

You can place a book between your knees and hold it there by pressing the knees together *(Fig. 6.7)*. This is useful if your knees have a tendency to separate on the downward movement.

Practising the posture a few inches from a wall *(Fig. 6.8)* corrects any tendency for your body to move too far forward.

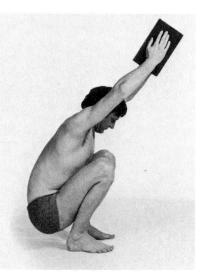

6.6

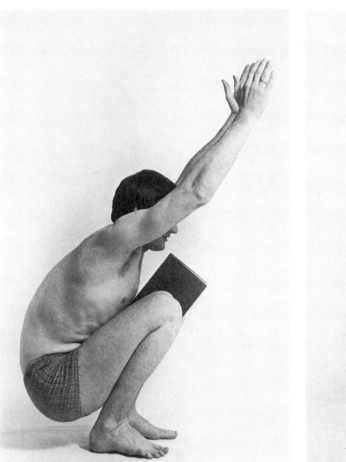

6.7

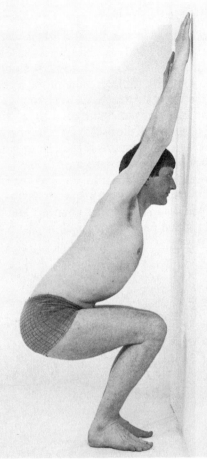

6.8

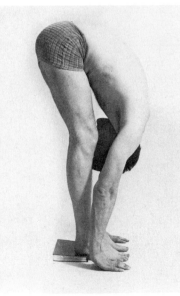

6.10

Uttanasana made easier

Similar modifications can be used in Uttanasana *(Fig. 6.9)*. By placing a book under your heels, the stretching in your legs is reduced *(Fig. 6.10)*. This is useful when the whole body is very stiff and the emphasis of the posture needs to be directed to your hips or your back.

Another modification with a similar effect is to bend your knees to reduce stretching in the legs. This produces more movement in your hips and back *(Fig. 6.11)*. When used dynamically, this modification helps the lower back to be worked more vigorously.

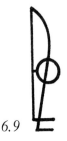

6.9

Uttanasana made harder

Placing a book between your hands will help work more on your arms, shoulders and back *(Fig. 6.12)*. You can also use this modification with one arm at a time *(Fig. 6.13)*. Placing a book under the front of your feet helps to intensify the stretching of the legs *(Fig. 6.14)*.

Another modification which will work your upper, middle and lower back involves placing your hands on a chair *(Fig. 6.15)*. The head is raised on inhalation and the back is arched. The same idea is used again in Fig. 6.16, but with the arms higher. Both these variations are very good for working the lower back.

By leaning against a wall *(Fig. 6.17)* you can reduce the movement of your hips while, at the same time, your lower back has to work more vigorously. The distance between your feet and the wall can be varied according to which part of your back needs to be worked.

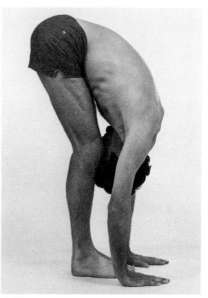

6.11

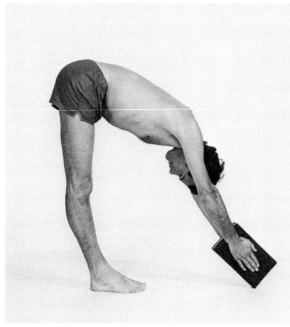

6.12

6.13

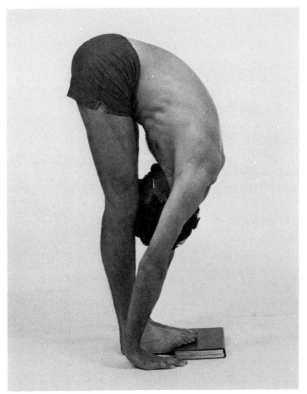

6.14

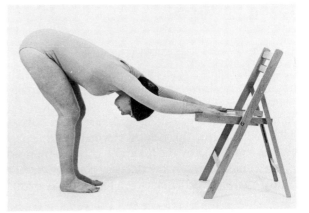

6.15

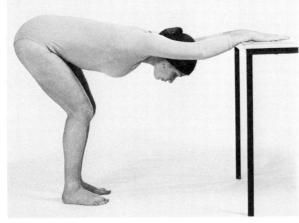

6.16

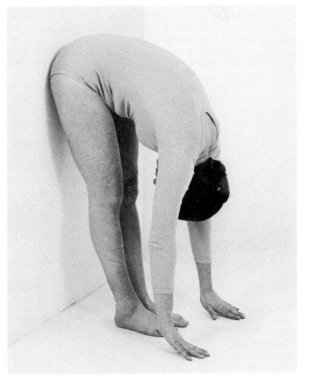

6.17

Lying postures

Savasana

Savasana *(Fig. 6.18)* appears a very simple posture but in some cases a number of modifications will be necessary to make it easier.

If you bend your legs, the lower part of the back, which is usually concave, becomes convex *(Fig. 6.19)*; if you have pain in your lower back you may find this helpful — when the knees are bent your lower back is supported by the floor and can rest more effectively.

You can achieve similar effects by placing your legs on a low stool or chair *(Fig. 6.20)* or by placing a folded towel or small cushion in the small of your back *(Fig. 6.21)*.

Other modifications to Savasana include putting a folded towel under your head when your chin has a tendency to stick up *(Fig. 6.22)*.

6.18

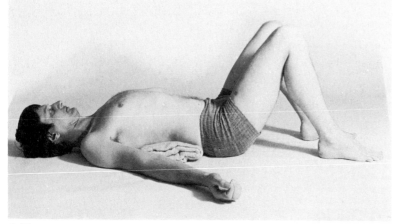

6.19

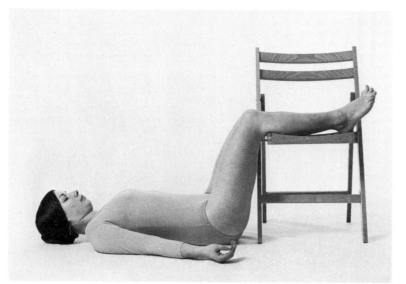

6.20

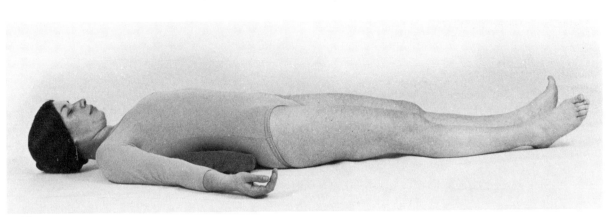

6.21

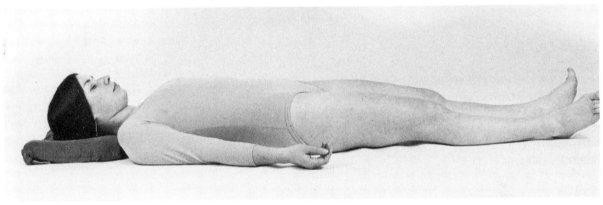

6.22

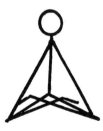

6.23

Sitting postures

Padmasana

Stiffness in your back, legs and knees, or hips will make Padmasana *(Fig. 6.23)* difficult for you and will result in a poor posture *(Fig. 6.24)*, where the back is slumped. You can improve the posture by placing a book or small cushion under your buttocks *(Fig. 6.25)*. Compare the difference between the two photographs. By raising the buttocks and changing the angle of the pelvis, the back becomes convex *(Fig. 6.25)*. The same is true in other sitting postures where the legs are crossed.

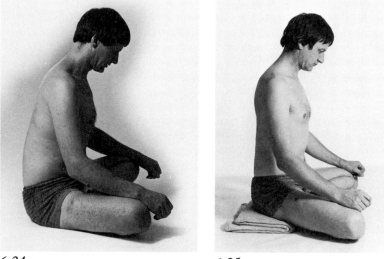

6.24   6.25

Tiryangmukha Ekapada Pascimatanasana

In Tiryangmukha Ekapada Pascimatanasana *(Fig. 6.26)*, stiffness in your hips, knees or ankles can prevent both buttocks from being placed on the floor. However, a small cushion or book under the buttock of the straight leg *(Figs. 6.27 and 6.28)* will help to keep your buttocks and hips level.

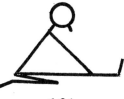

6.26

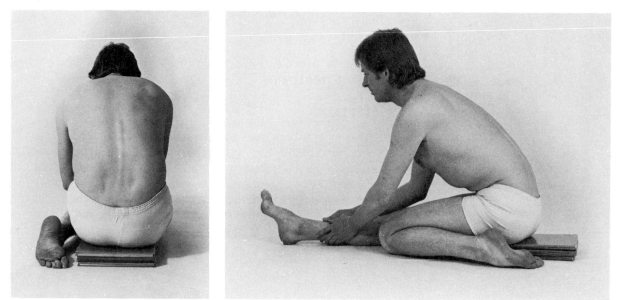

6.27   6.28

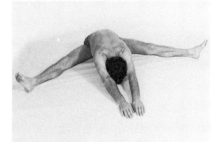

6.29

Upavista Konasana

Upavista Konasana *(Fig. 6.29)* can be modified in several ways. As in Padmasana, a book or cushion under the buttocks will change the angle of your hips and make it easier to bend forward *(Fig. 6.30)*. You can obtain the opposite·effect by placing a support under your feet *(Fig. 6.31)*. This increases the stretching in your legs and works your lower back more intensely.

A book between your hands *(Fig. 6.32)* will work your upper back and shoulders more. You can make the posture easier by bending your knees and you can make it asymmetrical by placing one arm behind your back. *(Fig. 6.33)*.

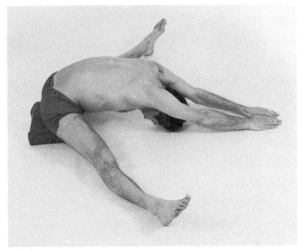

6.30

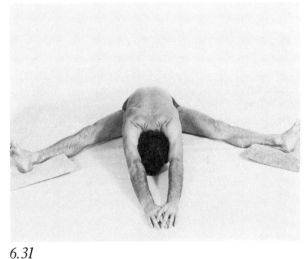

6.31

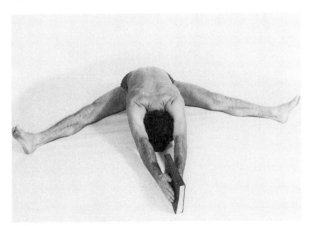

6.32

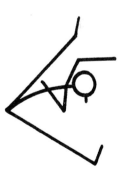

6.33

Where there is a lot of stiffness or weakness in the body you may have to modify the posture considerably. For example, with forward bends you can sit on a stool or chair *(Fig. 6.33)*.

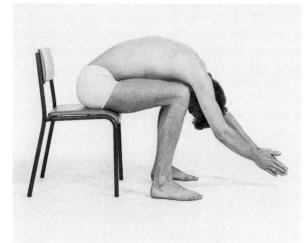

6.33a

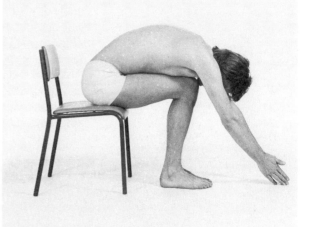

6.33b

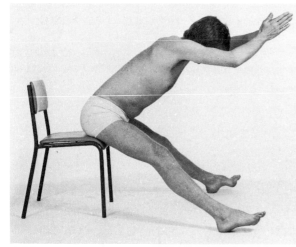

6.33c

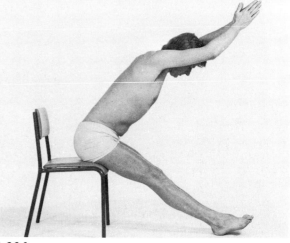

6.33d

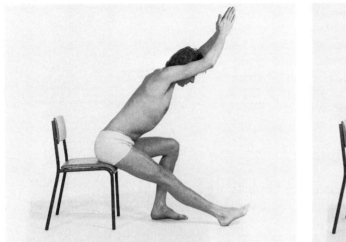

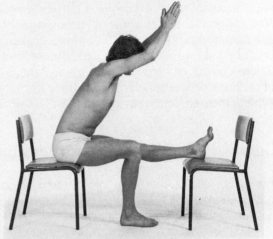

6.33e

6.33f

Modification when first learning Halasana

Modification of a posture is often necessary when first learning an asana. For example, in Halasana it is safer at first to place your feet on a chair (*Fig. 6.34*).

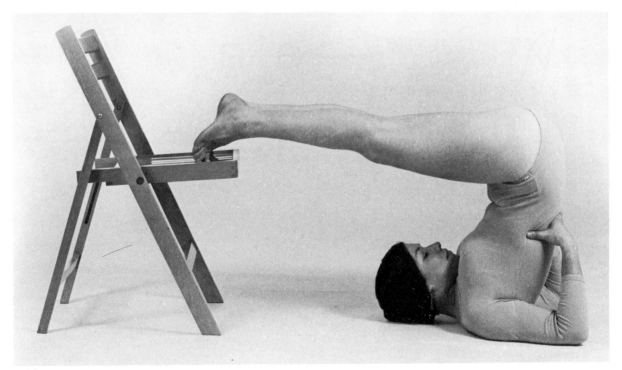

6.34

Modifications to find a student's weaknesses

The modification of asanas is also useful for a teacher who is attempting to find a student's weaknesses. By modifying a posture so that it becomes more strenuous, a particular weakness will become more noticeable. For example, if there is a problem in the student's neck or shoulders, a variation using a book in Tadasana *(Fig. 6.35)*will accentuate the problem. This can also be employed to clarify a student's breathing capacity; by working dynamically in Uttanasana with a book between the arms, the body has to work hard and any problem with inhalation or exhalation will be much easier to observe.

Combining different modifications

More than one modification can be used at once; for example, a modification for a forward bend may be used with a book under the buttocks and one in the hands.

Fig. 6.36 shows a Vinyasa with modification to work more on the lower back, and would be suitable for a student who is strong, but stiff. In contrast, the Vinyasa in Fig. 6.37 is an example of modifications which make postures easier for someone with a weak back.

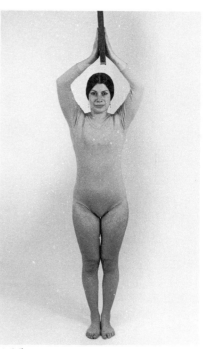

6.35

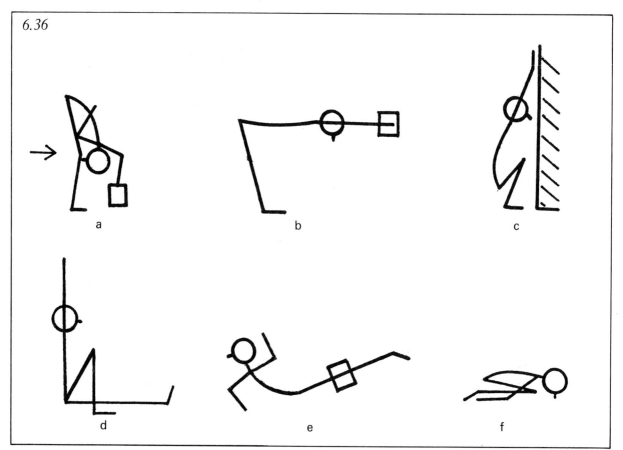

6.36

a

b

c

d

e

f

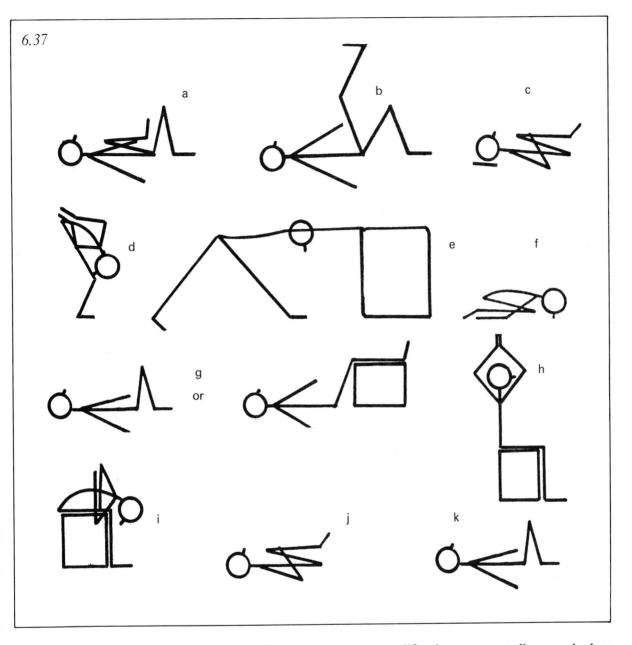

6.37

a   b   c

d   e   f

g
or

i   j   k

In all cases when you use modifications you must allow your body to be free. To tie or fix part of your body could be dangerous; if the modification is too strong, there is no way for your body to adapt to the strain and this could result in a muscle or ligament injury. Worse, a particular injury may not be immediately evident and the accumulated strain over a period of months or even years will only add to the damage.

Modifications and their permutations introduce a great variety to the classical postures and so help keep your practice creative and alive.

Questions and observations

1 Make a list of all the asanas in which a book can be held:
    a in between the hands;
    b in one hand;
    c placed between the knees.
2 What effects does modifying Dandasana by bending the knees *(Fig. 6.38)* have on:
    a your back?
    b your shoulders?
    c your breath?

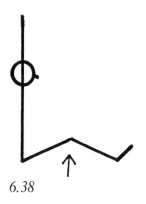

6.38

3 Modify Dvipada Pitham *(Fig. 6.39)* so that it works more on:
    a your shoulders;
    b your lower back;
    c your legs.

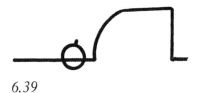

6.39

CHAPTER 7

Pascimatanasana

The purpose of this chapter is to illustrate how the principles of Vinyasa, counter-pose, variations, modifications and use of the breath in asanas, outlined in the previous chapters, affect one posture. It shows how refined and subtle an asana can be and how many different factors need to be considered when practising it.

Etymology

Pascimatanasana *(Fig. 7.1)* is one of the classical postures of yoga and is referred to in several of the yoga texts.

Pascima Literally means west. Traditionally in India, Yoga was practised facing the rising sun, with the front of the body (purva) facing the east and the back facing west. In this posture the west side or the back of the body and the back of the legs are stretched.

Tanu Means to spread.

Uttana Means to stretch up.

Asana Means seat, pose, posture.

In the *Hatha Yoga Pradipika* it is defined in this way: 'Stretch out both the legs on the ground without bending them, and having taken hold of the toes of the feet with the hands, place the forehead over the knees and rest thus.'

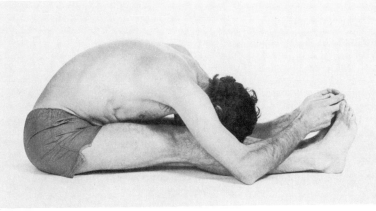

7.1

Technique

Dynamic

These instructions apply if you are supple and strong and used to forward bends. If your legs and back are stiff the modifications described on page 114 would be a more suitable way for you to work.

1 Sit in Dandasana *(Fig. 7.2a)*. Your legs should be straight in front of your body, your feet together and pointing upwards. Your spine should be straight, your chin down and your hands, palms down, on the floor, with your fingers pointing towards your feet. The weight of your body should be supported by your back and *not* your hands.

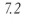

a

2 Inhaling, raise your arms above your body *(Fig. 7.2b)*.

IN
b

3 Exhaling, bend forward, with your arms in line with your body. Keep your arms back while moving forward. The forward movement should usually come from the *base* of your spine *(Fig. 7.2c)*.

c

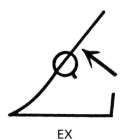

4 Inhaling, come up from the posture, lifting your arms first and arching your back and opening your chest *(Fig. 7.2d)*.

You can repeat the movement a number of times. Working dynamically is particularly useful when your body is stiff.

EX
d

Static

1 Inhaling, raise your arms above your head *(Fig. 7.3a)*.

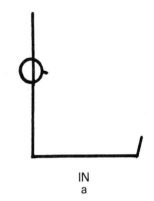

IN
a

2 Exhaling, bend halfway forward and take hold of the outside of your feet with your hands *(Fig. 7.3b)*.

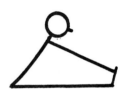

EX
b

3 Inhaling, stretch your spine and open your chest *(Fig. 7.3c)*.

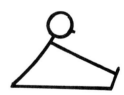

IN
c

4 Exhaling, bend forward, bending your elbows and stay for six to twelve breaths. Bending your elbows helps to relax your shoulders.

EX
d

Hints

1 Avoid trying to move too far into the posture. If your body is stiff, the movement should be stopped as soon as your back begins to curve. Your lower back should bend only in the last part of the movement.

2 Avoid hunching your shoulders *(Fig. 7.4)*. Keep them relaxed *(Fig. 7.5)*.

3 Do not use your arms too much to pull your body down towards your legs. Rather, work dynamically repeating the movement up and down, gradually extending it.

4 Be aware of the lower back and move as much as possible from this area.

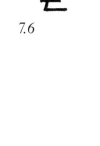

7.6

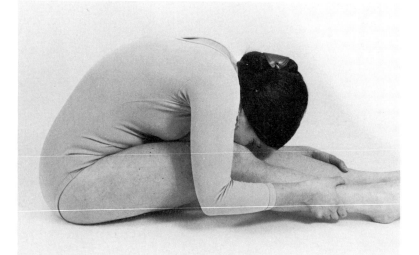

7.4

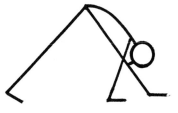

7.7

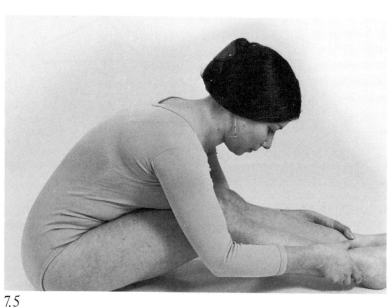

7.5

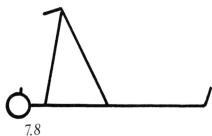

7.8

Preparation

The preparation for this asana, like other postures, will vary according to the individual. If you have stiff legs you will need to prepare in a different way from someone with supple legs and so the following suggestions are only of a very general nature.

Uttanasana *(Fig. 7.6)* is exactly the same movement as Pascimatanasana and will help prepare your legs, hips and back. The weight of your body helps the forward movement.

Parsva Uttanasana *(Fig. 7.7)* will help to stretch your legs more than Uttanasana and is useful if you find stiffness in your legs a problem with Pascimatanasana.

Supta Ekapada Padangusthasana *(Fig. 7.8)* will give a strong stretch to your legs. It also works your lower back to some extent.

Halasana *(Fig. 7.9)* works your lower back and also stretches your legs.

In some cases, Ardha Matsyendrasana *(Fig. 7.10)* and back bends also help work your lower back and loosen your hips in preparation for Pascimatanasana.

You might find that several modifications of forward bends can also be useful as preparation. Standing with one leg resting on a table and then bending forward helps stretch your legs *(Fig. 7.11)*. Sitting on a stool or chair with your legs bent *(Fig. 7.12)* helps prepare your back; conversely, your legs will be stretched more vigorously if they are straight *(Fig. 7.13)*. Another variation is with one foot on the floor and the other on a chair, as in Fig. 7.14.

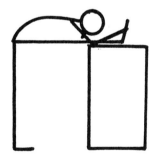

7.9

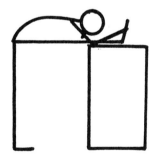

7.10

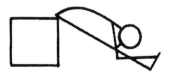

7.11

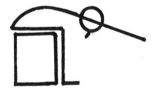

7.12

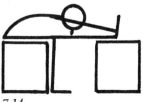

7.13

7.14

Counter-poses

There are several possible counter-poses for Pascimatanasana and the choice will depend on your individual needs, although if Pascimatanasana is a comfortable posture you may not need any counter-posture at all.

Catuspadapitham *(Fig. 7.15)* will work on your legs and hips. Purvattanasana *(Fig. 7.16)* is useful only if your hips are supple and your back can be arched. If this is not possible, there will not be enough movement in your body to allow the counter-posture to be effective.

Dvipada Pitham *(Fig. 7.17)* works your back, legs and also your shoulders and arms, although Apanasana *(Fig. 7.18)* may be necessary before Dvipada Pitham if you have held Pascimatanasana for a long time, or find it a demanding pose. In these cases moving from Pascimatanasana directly to Dvipada Pitham would be too strong.

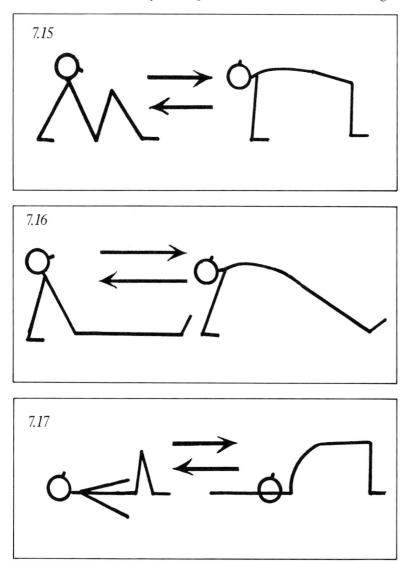

7.15

7.16

7.17

7.18

If you have a particularly stiff back, Cakravakasana *(Fig. 7.19)* may also be necessary as a counter-pose.

For stiff legs Apanasana *(Fig. 7.20)*, worked dynamically, is a useful counter-pose to help remove the negative effects of the main posture.

When there is considerable stiffness in the back, the counter-posture can be introduced halfway through the pose *(Fig. 7.21)*.

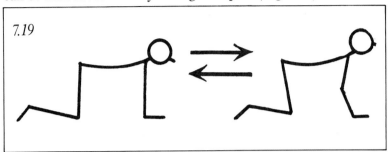

7.19

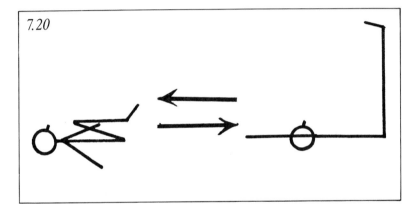

7.20

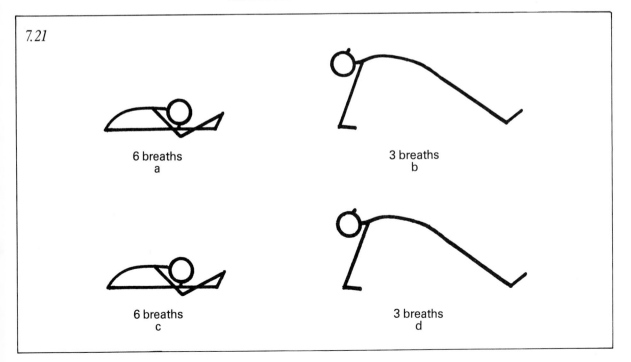

7.21

6 breaths
a

3 breaths
b

6 breaths
c

3 breaths
d

Examples of Vinyasas

1 Figure 7.22 shows a Vinyasa for a general class.
2 Figure 7.23 shows a Vinyasa for stiff legs.

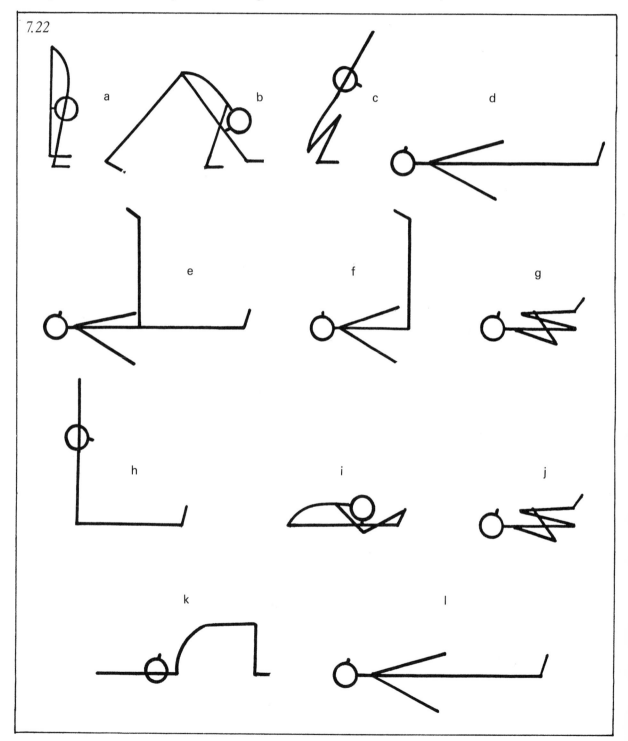

7.22

a b c d e f g h i j k l

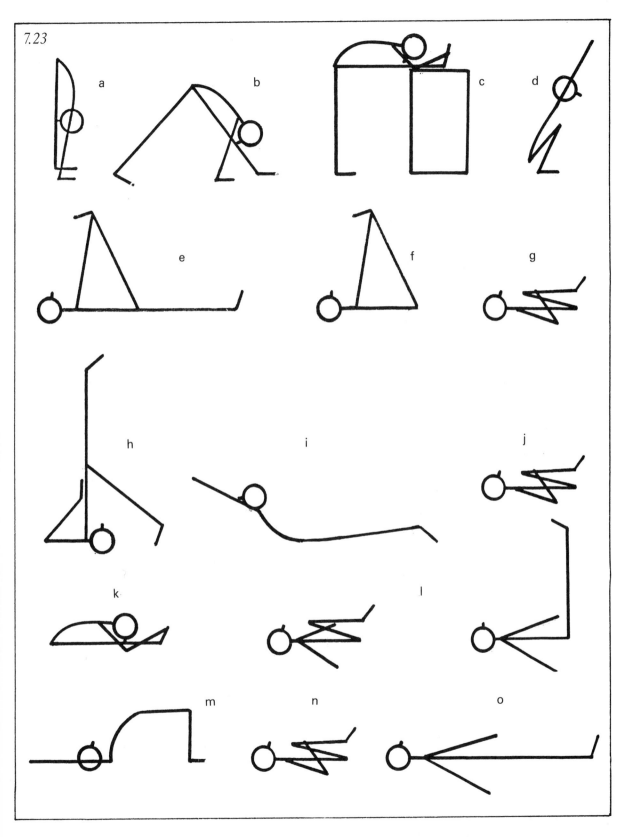

3 Figure 7.24 shows a Vinyasa for a stiff lower back.

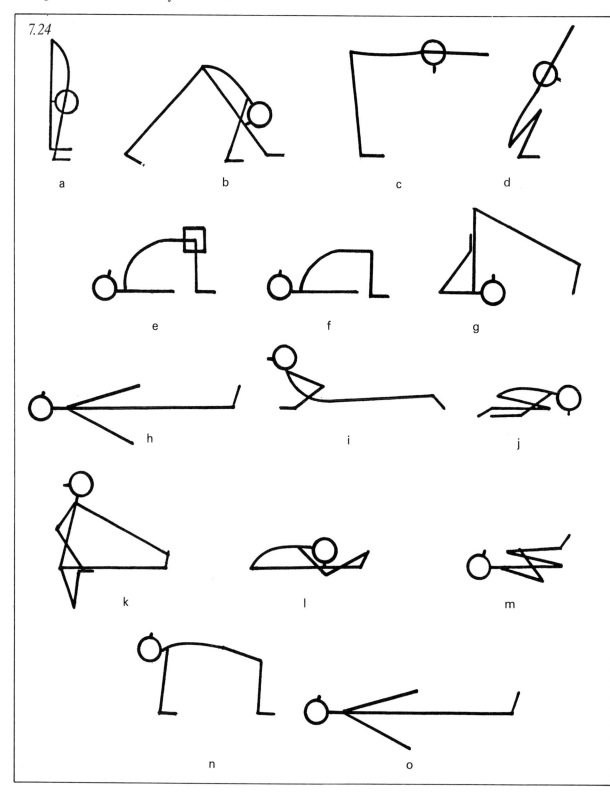

7.24

a b c d

e f g

h i j

k l m

n o

Pascimatanasana can itself be used as preparation in a Vinyasa for more difficult postures such as Upavista Konasana *(Fig. 7.25)*. Tiryangmukha Ekapada Pascimatanasana *(Fig. 7.26)* Krauncasana *(Fig. 7.27)* and Mahamudra *(Fig. 7.28)*.

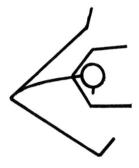

7.25

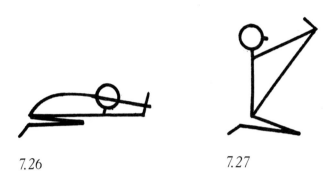

7.26   *7.27*

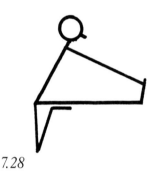

7.28

Variations on Pascimatanasana

Pascimatanasana has a large number of variations, each of which has a different effect on the body and the breath. It is very difficult to say exactly *what* the effect of a variation will be because it varies a great deal from one person to another. The different hand and arm positions possible in Pascimatanasana can considerably influence the effects of the posture.

Figure 7.29 shows the classical posture as described in the *Hatha Yoga Pradipika*.

Holding the outside edges of your feet works more along the sides of your legs and allows more movement in your back. This forward stretch can be intensified by interlocking your fingers across the soles *(Fig. 7.30)*. Turning your palms out has a similar effect but also works the wrist joint *(Fig. 7.31)*. Holding one wrist with your hand further increases the downward stretch of the pose *(Fig. 7.32)*.

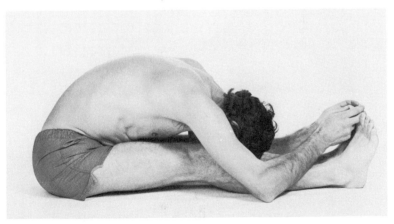

7.29

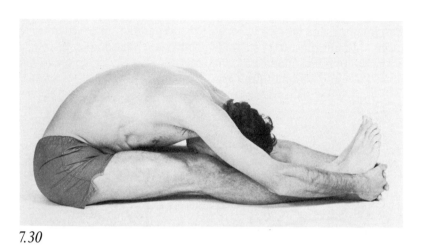

7.30

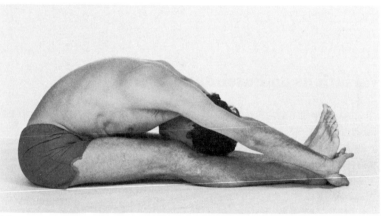

7.31

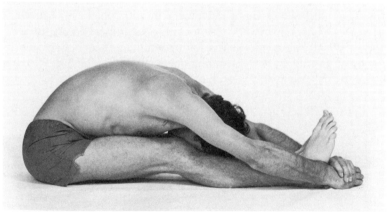

7.32

Another variation where the hands hold the feet has them on top of your feet *(Fig. 7.33)*. This tends to stretch the back of your legs more and also increases the stretch on your ankle joint.

Crossing the arms, so that your left hand holds your right foot and your right hand your left foot, often increases the stretch on your upper back *(Fig. 7.34)*.

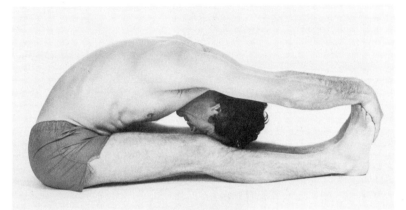

7.33

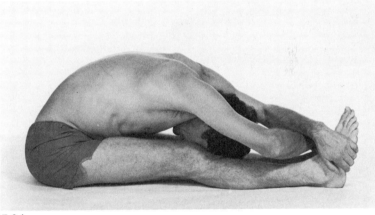

7.34

It is not essential that your hands hold your feet. When they do not, your body cannot be pulled into the pose and the forward movement has to come more from your back *(Fig. 7.35)*. With your hands on the floor, again your body cannot be pulled into the posture and your back has to work more to get into the posture *(Fig. 7.36)*.

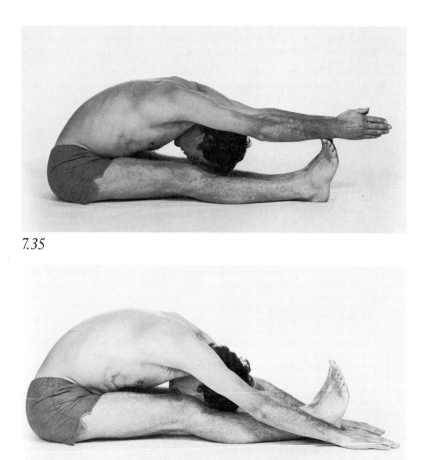

7.35

7.36

A simpler variation, with the arms bent, is useful if your shoulders are tense *(Fig. 7.37)*. You can also keep your shoulders and upper back relaxed by having your palms together with your arms bent *(Fig. 7.38)*.

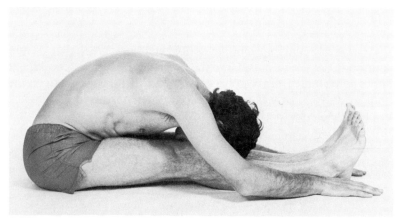

7.37

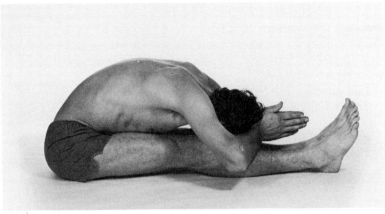

7.38

A more difficult variation has the arms at right-angles to the body *(Fig. 7.39)*. The forward-bending movement is harder because the weight of your arms cannot be used to help bring your body forward.

A variation combining different arm positions *(Fig. 7.40)* is often helpful to correct an imbalance in your back or shoulders.

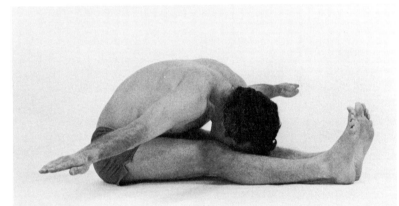

7.39

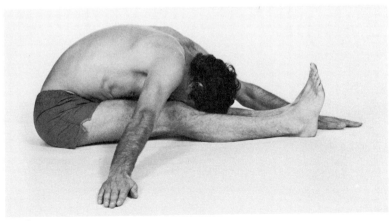

7.40

Keeping your arms behind your back *(Fig. 7.41)* helps prevent rounding the shoulders, a very common mistake when first learning the pose. Another variation is with your arms stretched behind your back *(Fig. 7.42)*, while placing your palms together makes the position even harder *(Fig. 7.43)*.

The variation in *(Fig. 7.44)* combines the advantages of working asymmetrically with work on the shoulders.

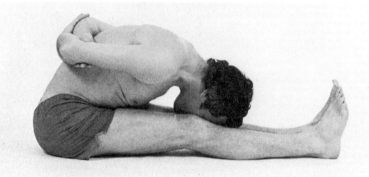

7.41

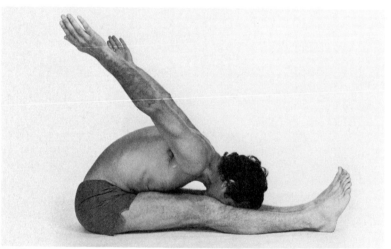

7.42

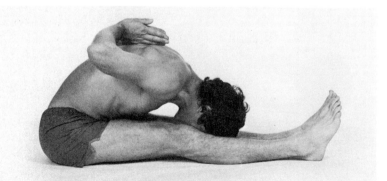

7.43

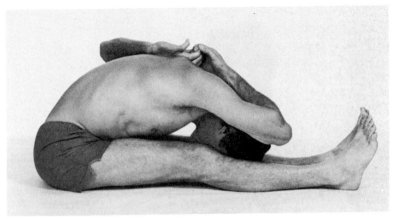

7.44

Modifications of Pascimatanasana

Pascimatanasana can be modified in many ways, either to make the posture easier or harder, or to work a particular area of the body, usually the back, more effectively. Generally it is more important to modify the posture so it is easier because if your body is stiff the forward movement is restricted and this often results in your back curving and your shoulders being tense and hunched *(see Fig. 7.4).*

Modifications to make the posture easier

Bending your knees is one of the simplest modifications *(Fig. 7.45).* The stretching effect on your legs is lost but far more movement is possible in your back and hips. You might try using this modification for six breaths before working with your legs straight.

Another simple but effective modification is to restrict the forward bend to a few inches by placing your hands on your legs below the knees *(Fig. 7.46).* This position is very effective for working the lower back. Bending further forward and holding the ankles *(Fig. 7.47)* is another modification and alters the area of the back which is worked.

If your back and legs are stiff, a towel placed around your feet will help you to keep your back straight in the posture *(Fig. 7.48).* The forward movement can be made by gently pulling on the towel, although you should avoid pulling too much as this can cause strain.

Placing a small stool or thick book under your buttocks opens the hip joints and allows for more rotation in the pelvis *(Fig. 7.49).*

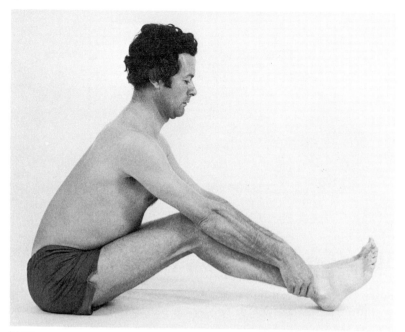

7.45

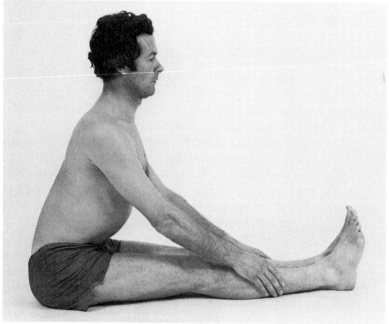

7.46

110

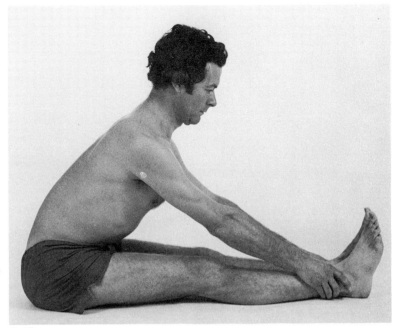

7.47

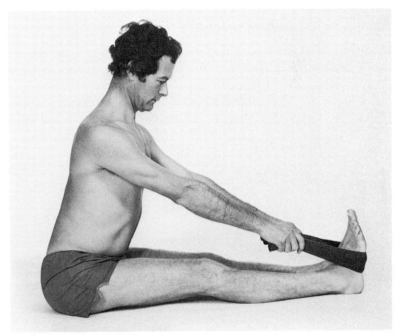

7.48

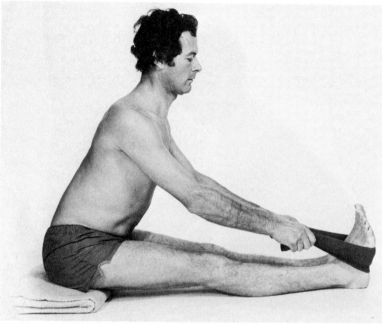

7.49

Modifications which intensify the posture

Placing your feet on a book or on a stool restricts the movement of your hips so that your back has to work more for your body to come forward *(Fig. 7.50)*.

A book between your hands works the arms, shoulders and upper back more, and is very effective for strengthening arms and back *(Fig. 7.51)*.

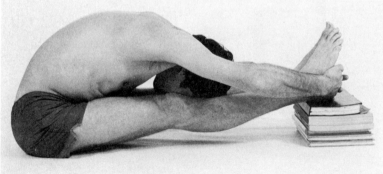

7.50

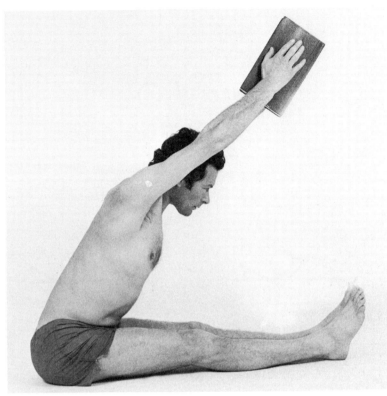

7.51

Working with the breath

Pascimatanasana is a forward-bending posture and therefore longer exhalation than inhalation is usually more appropriate, although this is not always the case.

While staying statically in the posture a fairly easy ratio is 1:1½, e.g. 8:0:12:0, or 1:2, e.g. 8:0:16:0. Once you can hold the posture comfortably for twelve to twenty-four long breaths (5—10 minutes) without the quality of your breath deteriorating, retention of the breath can gradually be introduced.

If you can maintain 8:0:16:0 for twelve breaths, 6:0:12:4 or 6:0:12:6 should be possible. Retention of the breath helps the forward movement and increases the effect of the posture.

Working dynamically in the posture, so that your body comes partly or all the way up, allows the breath to be held after the inhalation and/ or after the exhalation *(Fig. 7.52)*. Alternatively, the exhalation could be longer and the retention after exhalation reduced or completely eliminated *(Fig. 7.53)*. Many other ratios are possible in this pose and the choice of which one depends upon your needs and the advice of your teacher.

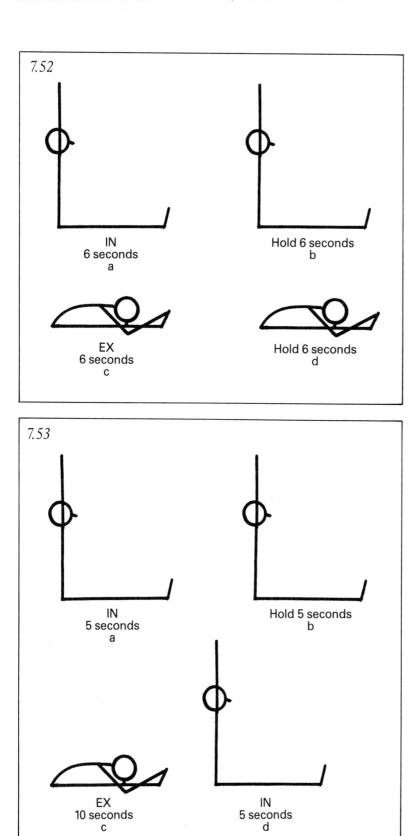

7.52

IN
6 seconds
a

Hold 6 seconds
b

EX
6 seconds
c

Hold 6 seconds
d

7.53

IN
5 seconds
a

Hold 5 seconds
b

EX
10 seconds
c

IN
5 seconds
d

Questions and observations

1 Compare the Vinyasas in Figs. 7.54 and 7.55.

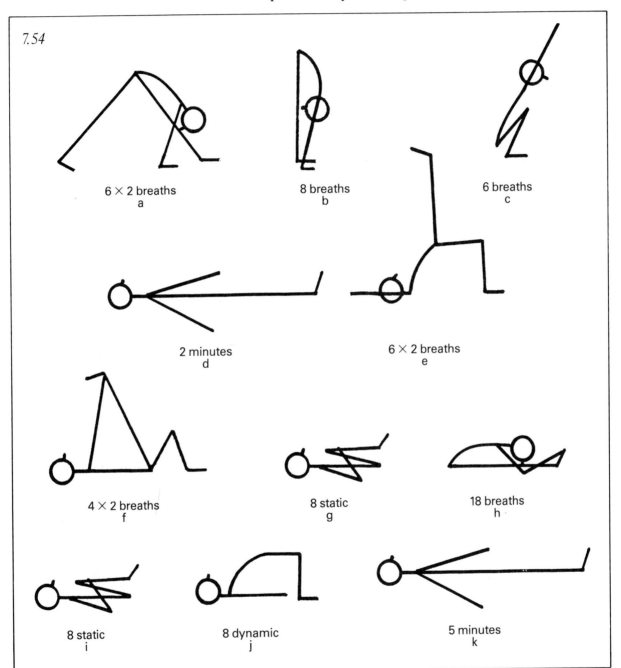

7.54

6 × 2 breaths
a

8 breaths
b

6 breaths
c

2 minutes
d

6 × 2 breaths
e

4 × 2 breaths
f

8 static
g

18 breaths
h

8 static
i

8 dynamic
j

5 minutes
k

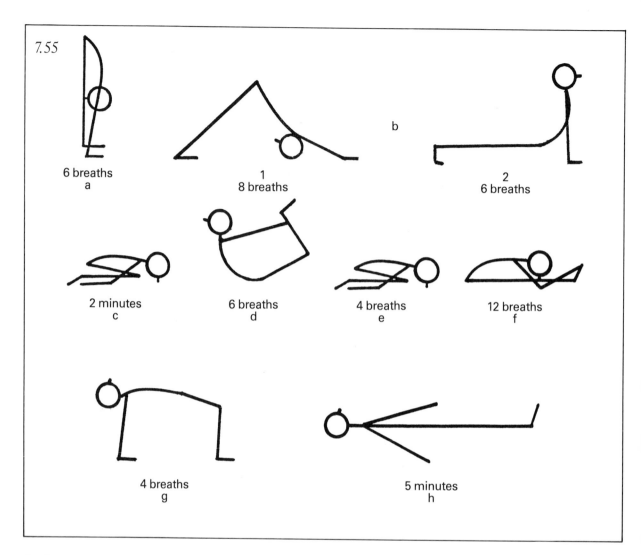

7.55

6 breaths
a

1
8 breaths

b

2
6 breaths

2 minutes
c

6 breaths
d

4 breaths
e

12 breaths
f

4 breaths
g

5 minutes
h

2 Compare working in Pascimatanasana for twelve breaths with a
1:0:1:0 and 1:0:2:0 ratio. Use the same Vinyasa for the preparation.

3 Observe the effects of the variations in Fig. 7.56. on:
a your lower back;
b shoulders;
c degree of forward movement.

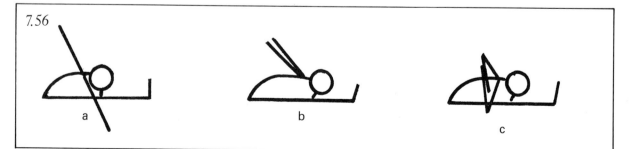

7.56

a

b

c

CHAPTER 8

Observation and Analysis

Observing and analysing your own practice are two of the most important elements in developing a creative attitude towards your practice. Without an awareness of how you are moving, of the quality and sound of your breath, and of the areas of stiffness in different parts of your body, your practice will be much less effective, both physically and mentally. Once you have the ability to observe your practice you can choose the variations, modifications of postures, particular breathing ratios and counter-poses which will be most suitable to your own individual needs. You can develop this ability not only by carefully watching your body and breath in the posture but also by watching other students practising postures.

However, while self-observation is helpful, it can only take you so far and you will still need the advice of a teacher who is specifically trained to observe and analyse a student's practice. Observation and analysis play an absolutely vital part in the effective teaching of yoga. Without the correct use of these two fundamental tools, a yoga teacher can sometimes do more harm than good. If, for example, a pupil has very stiff knees and the teacher fails to observe this and teaches Padmasana (*Fig. 8.1*), he can cause severe damage. Failure to observe the mental condition of a pupil can have equally harmful results. A pupil suffering from tension might need a very gentle practice, with plenty of lying postures; if he was given a predominance of standing postures, particularly at the beginning of the practice, it could easily increase the tension already present. It is possible to assess a student's physical condition and, to some extent, his mental state, by watching him perform a number of simple asanas.

8.1

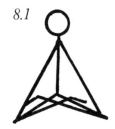

Some of the main features you should look for in your own practice are as follows.

1 The quality of your concentration.
2 The quality of your breath.
3 The quality of your coordination.
4 The degree of your strength and suppleness; for instance, are you:
   a strong and supple;
   b strong and stiff;
   c weak and supple; or
   d weak and stiff?
5 Do you have particular areas of restriction, stiffness and weakness, such as a stiff hip or leg, weakness in your back and restricted movement of your head?

Observation and teaching

Teachers within this tradition often use some of the postures in Fig. 8.2 to observe and diagnose a student's practice. While these postures are useful from a teacher's point of view, they are not meant to be practised by a student without supervision.

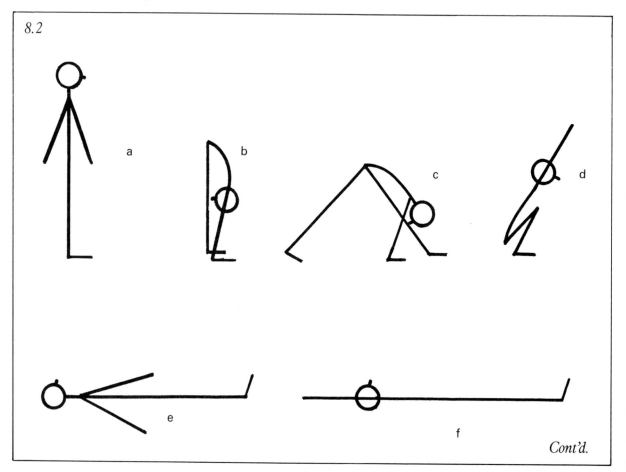

8.2

Cont'd.

118

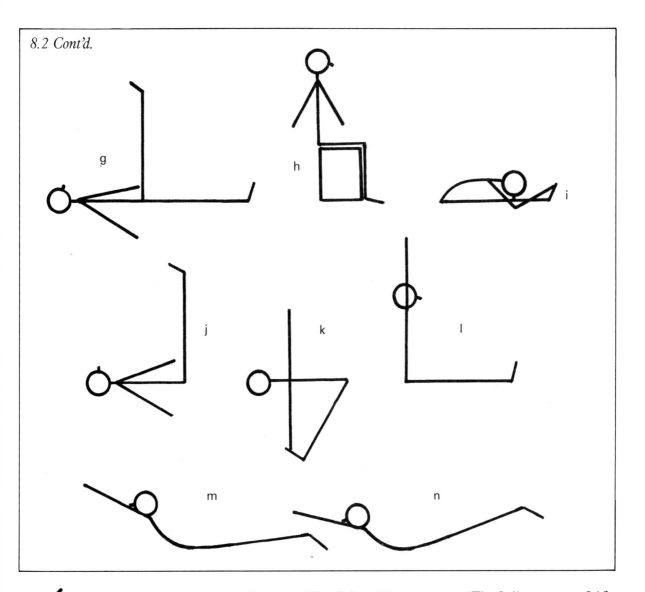

8.2 Cont'd.

g

h

i

j

k

l

m

n

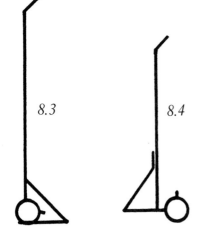

8.3

8.4

Sirsasana *(Fig. 8.3)* and Sarvangasana *(Fig. 8.4)* are very useful for observation, provided the student is ready to practise them. Both postures can often reveal imbalances on one side of the body, not easily observed in other postures. Sarvangasana is also very helpful for observing the breathing capacity because it restricts the movement of the chest.

The remaining part of this chapter has been written primarily from the point of view of helping a yoga teacher. However, many of the points raised and the general concept of observation will be of use to you in helping you to improve your practice.

The ability of a teacher to observe accurately is greatly influenced by the number of students in a class. Obviously, if the class is very large it is impossible for the teacher to watch each student closely. This may be one of the reasons why in India asanas and Pranayama have been taught either individually or in very small groups. It is then possible for the teacher to observe very precisely the mental and physical make-up of *each* student and to adapt the teaching to individual needs.

Mental observation

It is now an accepted principle of psychology that the way people think has a profound effect on their bodies and that the body has a profound effect on the mind. Mental problems often manifest themselves physically, and vice versa. Because of this deep interrelationship, it is not possible to separate the two. However, initially, it may be useful to consider the two apart.

Each one of us presents to the world a façade, projecting an image which is usually very different from our real personality. It is clear that if a teacher is really to help a student he must attempt to see beyond this external level. Although a good deal of information can be observed in the first class or two, it naturally takes time, even in individual classes, really to get to know a pupil. With a group class, even of six to eight people, it is obviously more difficult and takes even longer.

Teachers can make many useful observations about their students in the first class by noting simple things, such as how students walk into the room, whether they appear to be calm and relaxed or tense, how they move, or even how they shake hands. In either individual or small group classes it is useful to spend some time talking to the students to get to know them and to establish why they have come to a class and what they expect from it.

Concentration

Concentration plays a primary role in all yoga disciplines. Concentration is defined as the ability of the mind to become absorbed in one idea, so that all other ideas are automatically excluded. One of the most important aspects of the practice of asanas and Pranayama is that the mind should be totally absorbed in the practice.

It is fairly easy to observe how much concentration a student has in his practice by noting whether his movements are made with care and attention or are performed in an automatic and rather dead fashion. With concentration, a particular quality comes into the way a student moves.

A student who is supple might be able to do an asana beautifully but if he is not concentrating on the posture he is NOT practising yoga. On the other hand, a student who is very stiff and can only bend a short way but who is completely concentrated in the practice, IS practising yoga.

Physical observation

Obvious points to observe are age and general build. Different physiques will make a considerable difference to how a student works in particular asanas. For example, someone with a long body and neck would have to be very careful about doing Sirsasana *(Fig. 8.5)*; someone who is short and stocky could have difficulty with twisting asanas; and short arms will tend to make Pascimatanasana *(Fig. 8.6)* difficult.

The body is extremely complex. Its condition is subject to many variables and an almost infinite number of permutations, such as stiff hips, loose hips, stiff back, etc. To help simplify this very complex structure it might be useful first to consider the back and neck.

A good deal of information about the back can be gathered simply by observing, sideways on, how a student stands in Samasthiti.

The normal shape of the back has four curves, two primary (a and b in *Fig. 8.7*) and two secondary. This natural shape gives the spine a great deal more strength. By looking at a student's back from the side (the use of a wall helps measure the shape more accurately) it is possible to note the shape of the back, and whether the curves are normal or are more or less pronounced.

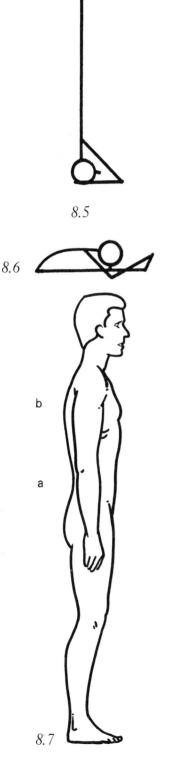

8.5

8.6

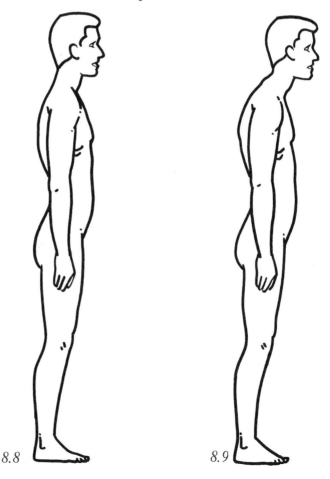

b

a

8.7

8.8

8.9

121

In Fig. 8.8 the lower back is hollowed and the upper back slightly bent forward. A pronounced curve in the lower back *(Fig. 8.9)* is often compensated for by a pronounced curve in the upper back. There are, however, exceptions to this, as in Fig. 8.10, where the upper back is fairly flat. In Fig. 8.11 there is a pronounced curve of the upper back and in Fig. 8.12 both the curves are very slight.

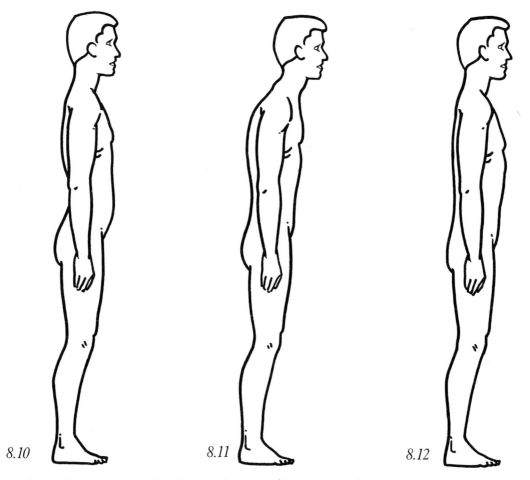

8.10   *8.11*   *8.12*

It is also useful to view a student from both sides and to compare the distance between each shoulder and a wall. If these are not equal it would indicate that there is a twist in the spine *(Fig. 8.13)*. (The heels, of course, must be parallel to the wall.)

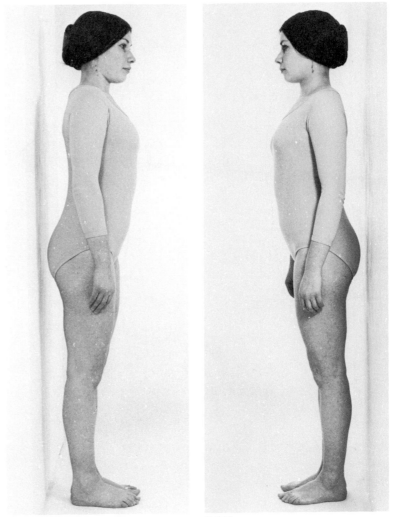

8.13a 8.13b

Visual observation of the back from behind can often reveal whether there are any side curves. Where the back is straight, the groove which runs up from the bottom of the back to the top will be straight *(Fig. 8.14)* and the whole body will be symmetrical. The hips and shoulders will be parallel and the space between the legs will be symmetrical. However, where there is a side curve in the spine the groove in the back will not be straight *(Fig. 8.15)* and the rest of the body will be affected. Shoulders and hips will be at an angle and the *shapes* in between the arm and the body will be uneven. If the curve in the spine is very marked it is easy to observe, but if it is only a small curve it is more difficult to detect.

Raising the arms to shoulder height *(Fig. 8.16)* will help to accentuate the imbalance as the arms will have a tendency to come up in an uneven fashion. However, this is in itself only an indication and is not sufficient to diagnose a curved spine, as any imbalance could equally well be caused by a problem in the shoulders.

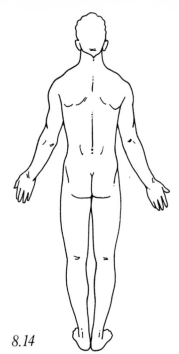

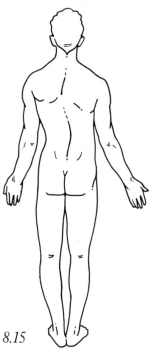

8.14

8.15

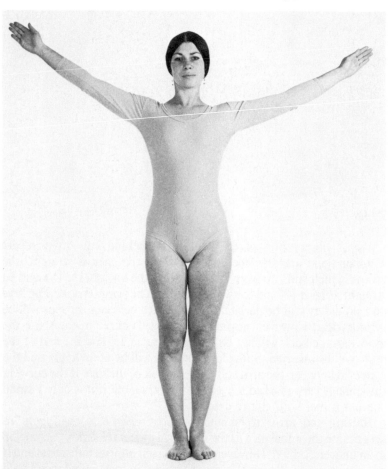

8.16

124

Observation of the body in Uttanasana

Uttanasana is an excellent posture for discovering many things about a student's body. It works on all parts of the back and legs and, with its many variations (see Chapter 6), a great deal more can be learnt about other parts of the body.

If the back is observed carefully as the body moves forward in the asana and back up again, it is possible to see those areas in the back which are flexible and those which are stiff. The spine is made up of thirty-three separate vertebrae, twenty-four of which are movable joints. Quite often some of these joints lose their mobility so that a number of them form a block. When the body moves in an asana these blocks can be noticed and it is important that the teacher observes them so that the student's practice can be modified accordingly. Fig. 8.17 shows some stiffness in the lower part of the back, while Fig. 8.18 shows the stiffness more in the upper back.

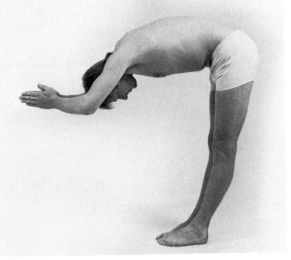

8.18

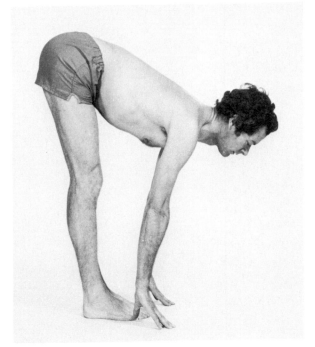

8.17

The forward-bending movement will also be influenced by other areas of stiffness in the body such as stiff legs. A further point for teachers to observe is how much backward movement there is in the hips *(Fig. 8.19)*. It is impossible to move into the posture without some backward movement *(Fig. 8.19a)*; however, a lot of movement *(Fig. 8.19b)* would indicate weakness in the back, as the body attempts to compensate by shifting the centre of gravity and so reduces the amount of work the back has to do. A student with very loose hips has a tendency to do this in Uttanasana.

Observing the movement from the front *(Fig. 8.20)* will often reveal problems which cannot be seen from the side. If there is an imbalance in the back it can be observed by comparing the shape of one side of the back with the other.

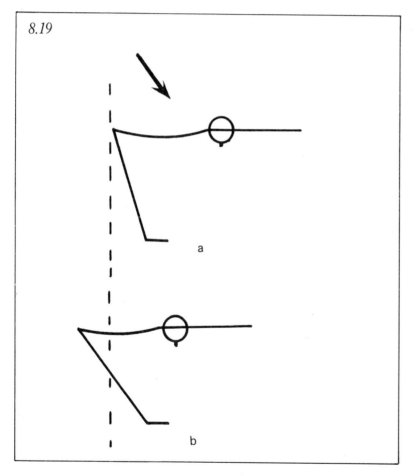

8.19

a

b

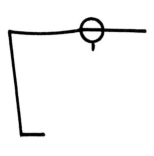

8.21

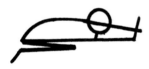

8.22

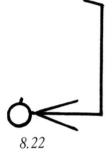

8.23

Legs and hips

Stiffness in the legs can be seen in a tendency either to bend at the knees and/or for the legs to shake, particularly in the variation Ardha Uttanasana *(Fig. 8.21)* or Urdhva Prasrta Padasana *(Fig. 8.22)*.

The mobility of the hips is a little more difficult to observe. If the hips are very stiff the movement will be very restricted. When the movement is very easy, and there is no stretching of the legs or the back, the pupil's hip joints will be very loose. For an accurate assessment of the flexibility of the hip joints, other postures such as Tiryangmukha Ekapada Pascimatanasana *(Fig. 8.23)* will be necessary.

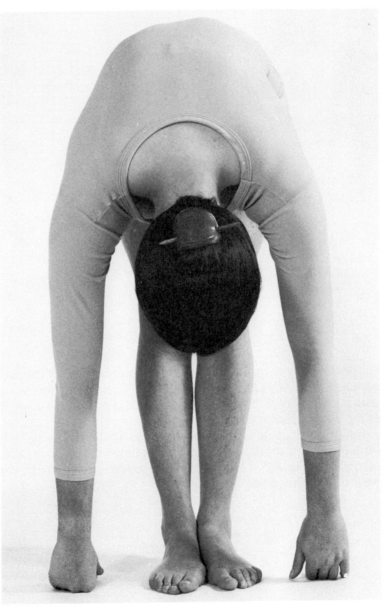

8.20

Asymmetrical asanas are useful in observation because they work on different sides of the body, enabling a comparison to be made between the two sides. In Parsva Uttanasana *(Fig. 8.24)* it is possible to compare the mobility of the right and left hips, the flexibility and strength of the leg muscles and of each side of the back. Where, for example, one leg is stiffer than another, the stretching in the stiffer leg will be greater and this may be detected by shaking or by a difficulty in maintaining balance. Where this is very pronounced the back heel may come up off the ground *(Fig. 8.25)*. Similarly, where one side of the back is stiffer than the other, the forward movement will be less on that side, and where one hip is stiffer the movement on that side will be reduced and the leg may have a tendency to shake.

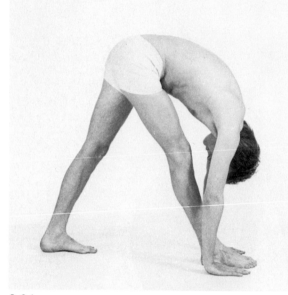

8.24

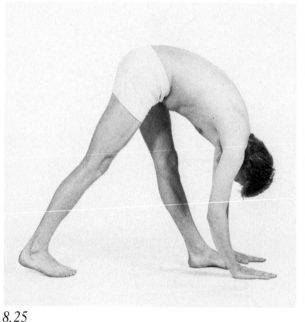

8.25

The flexibility of the hip will need to be assessed in other postures such as Utkatasana *(Fig. 8.26)*. This asana is also useful for noting both the flexibility of the hips, knees and ankle joints, and the strength of the legs and, particularly, of the thighs.

If the ankle joint or achilles tendon is very stiff it prevents the body from performing the downward movement unless the heels are raised off the floor *(Fig. 8.27)*. This is particularly common with women who wear high-heeled shoes.

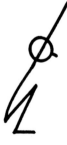

8.26

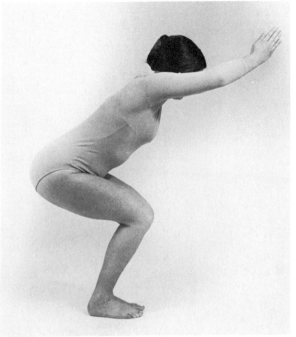

8.28

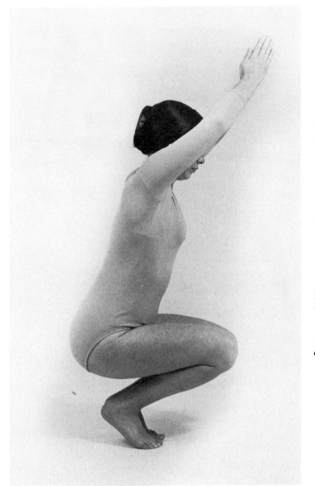

8.27

Observing the downward and upward movement of the back again gives an indication of its strength and suppleness. By keeping the arms above the head and not letting the body move too far forward the upper back is worked strongly. Many students, unconsciously attempting to avoid this by leaning forward, may lift the hips and lower back first *(Fig. 8.28)*.

Useful observations can also be made from the front as to how students move up and down in Utkatasana. It is quite common for there to be a sideways movement of the hips, particularly at about the halfway point *(Fig. 8.29)*. This could indicate that one hip is looser than the other and/or that there is an imbalance in the back and/or a weakness in one knee. The legs can also spread apart when going down *(Fig. 8.30)* or the knees can come together *(Fig. 8.31)*. This often happens when the legs are weak.

Because Utkatasana is a demanding posture it is very useful when used dynamically in order to assess a student's stamina. To be able to repeat the posture and keep control of the breath for between eight and twelve breaths requires a fair degree of strength.

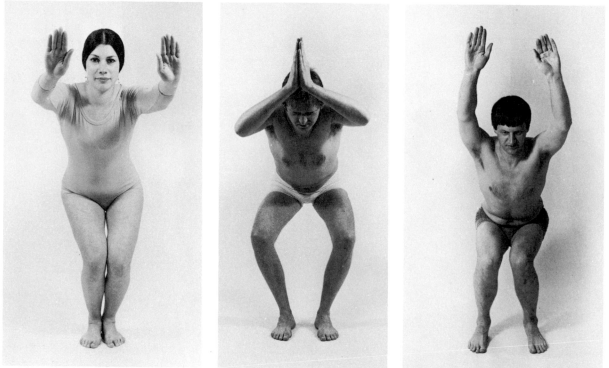

8.29   8.30   8.31

Lying postures

Savasana *(Fig. 8.32)* is a posture that can reveal a great deal about the student's body. A student with a symmetrical body will lie down straight, with the shoulders and hips parallel, as when standing, but where there is an imbalance, the hips and shoulders will be at an angle and the legs will tend to move to one side.

Where one hip has more outward rotation than the other, the foot of the leg with the loose hip will tend to fall closer to the floor *(Fig. 8.33)*.

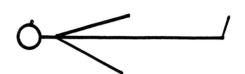

8.32

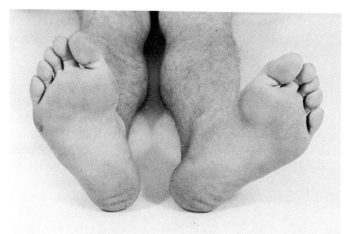

8.33

Supta Ekapada Prasrta Padasana *(Fig. 8.34)* is particularly useful in observing the flexibility and strength of the legs and stomach muscles. Where the upward-raising movement of one leg is restricted *(Fig. 8.35)* the cause is usually stiffness in the muscles of the back of the leg. This stiffness may be emphasised by shaking. It is useful to see if each leg can be raised to the same extent, or if one has more movement.

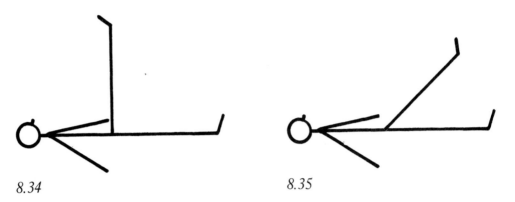

8.34   8.35

Where it is very easy for the leg to be raised to 90° or more *(Fig. 8.36),* the movement often comes from a very loose hip joint. If the leg is then lowered a little to approximately 80° or 60° and held for several breaths, many students will find this very difficult, and if the leg is weak it will begin to shake.

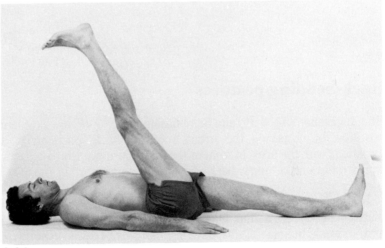

8.36

Raising both legs at the same time in Urdhva Prasrta Padasana *(Fig. 8.37)* and repeating the movement up and down is an excellent test for the strength of the stomach muscles and, to some extent, the back muscles. When the stomach muscles are weak they will tremble and it will be difficult to repeat the movement more than a few times. If the lower back is weak it will arch a lot during the movement *(Fig. 8.38)*. If the upper back is stiff there will be a tendency for the hands and arms to press against the floor for support and for the chin to rise up as the movement is repeated.

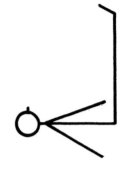

8.37

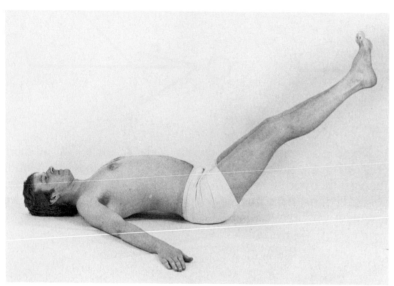

8.38

Back-bending postures

Bhujangasana *(Fig. 8.39)* and Salabhasana *(Fig. 8.40)* are excellent postures for observing the strength of the back, particularly if variations with the arms in front of the body are used. Bhujangasana works more on the upper back and Salabhasana more in the lower back.

In Bhujangasana, if it is possible for a student to raise the arms, head and upper body only a short way *(Fig. 8.41)*, the back is either very stiff and/or weak. In Salabhasana, if the legs can only be raised a short way *(Fig. 8.42)*, the lower back is weak. Other points to observe in Salabhasana are whether the legs remain together or apart, whether they both spread apart *(Fig. 8.43)* or whether one leg moves more than the other. These indicate looseness in one or both hips. It is important also to note whether the legs are straight or bent, and whether one leg is bent more than the other. If this is the case the heels will not be even *(Fig. 8.44)*.

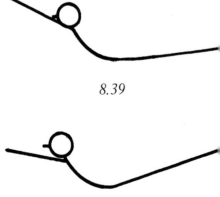

8.39

8.40

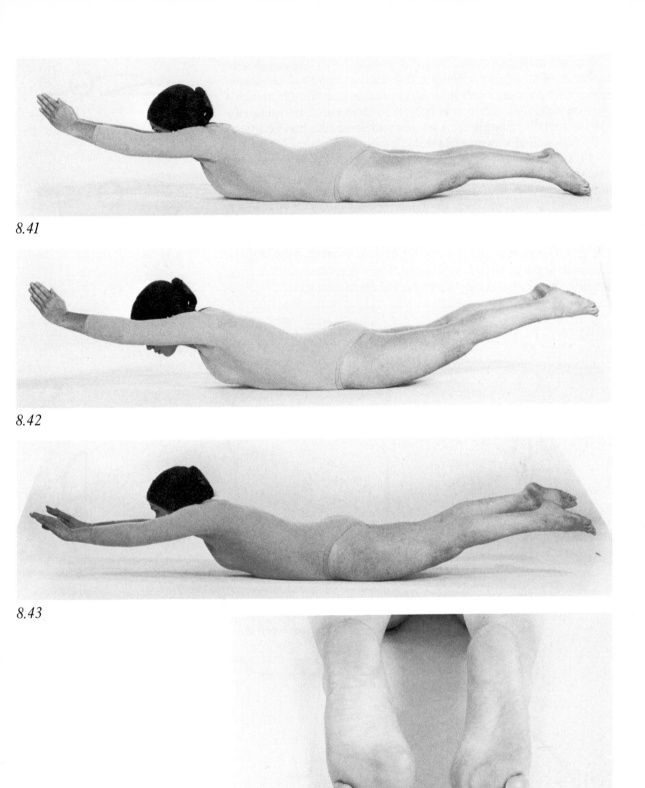

8.41

8.42

8.43

8.44

Because these two postures are demanding they are a valuable indication of the student's strength and stamina. Similar observations using other postures will help to obtain a clear idea of each student's physical condition. Often it is helpful to cross-check by using two asanas from the same group. A student with loose hips may be able to bend very well in Pascimatanasana, despite the fact that his back is very stiff. But Vajrasana *(Fig. 8.45)* with the arms in front of the body may show up more clearly the fact that the movement comes from the hips by making the stiffness in the back more apparent. An asymmetrical posture such as Janu Sirsasana *(Fig. 8.46)*, which restricts the movement of one hip at a time, shows more clearly the mobility of the back.

Fig. 8.47 is an example of notes taken on one student; it may help to illustrate the points already mentioned. These notes were taken during the first classes of a twenty-nine-year-old female student.

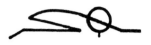

8.45

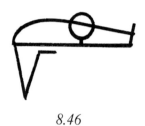

8.46

8.47

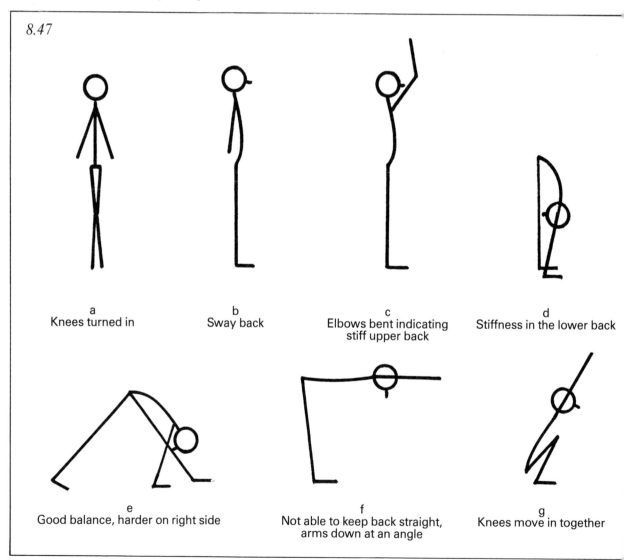

a
Knees turned in

b
Sway back

c
Elbows bent indicating stiff upper back

d
Stiffness in the lower back

e
Good balance, harder on right side

f
Not able to keep back straight, arms down at an angle

g
Knees move in together

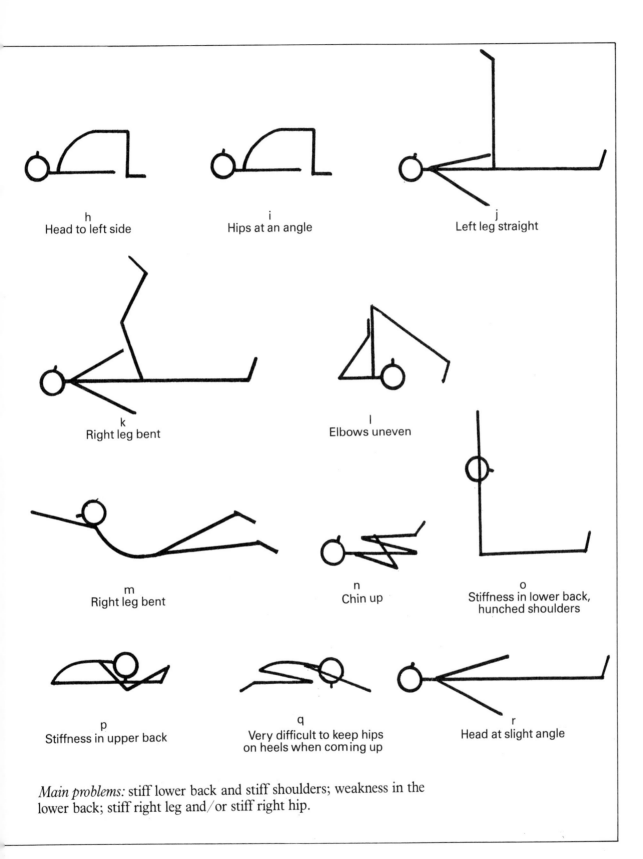

h
Head to left side

i
Hips at an angle

j
Left leg straight

k
Right leg bent

l
Elbows uneven

m
Right leg bent

n
Chin up

o
Stiffness in lower back,
hunched shoulders

p
Stiffness in upper back

q
Very difficult to keep hips
on heels when coming up

r
Head at slight angle

Main problems: stiff lower back and stiff shoulders; weakness in the lower back; stiff right leg and/or stiff right hip.

Observation of breathing

Within this tradition great emphasis is put on observing the way a student breathes. Notice which part of the chest is used and how much expansion takes place in the upper or middle chest and the abdomen. The quality of the breath is also noted to see whether it is controlled and even or irregular and rough, and whether control of the breath is better on the inhalation or exhalation and at the beginning őr the end of the breath.

Different postures affect differently the way the lungs function. By observing how the breath responds in the various asanas it is possible to get a clear indication not only of a student's breathing capacity, but also of where the breathing is weak and where it is strong.

The example in Fig. 8.48 shows notes made while observing the practice of a thirty-three-year-old man. The breath in Savasana (a) is quite long. The length of the breath will naturally become shorter with strenuous postures such as Uttanasana (c), but it drops a great deal more than would be expected in Trikonasana (d), Sarvangasana (j) and Ardha Matsyendrasana (m). The teacher diagnosed restriction in the upper chest and began working with postures and breathing ratios to increase the breathing capacity in this area.

Fig. 8.49 shows another example, of a twenty-seven-year-old man. In this example the breath is longer, particularly on the inhalation. However, the teacher noticed that the exhalation tended to be short. Normally one expects the exhalation to be longer than the inhalation, but in this case the inhalation and exhalation tended to be the same length, even in Pascimatanasana (n). Here the teacher recommended an emphasis on forward-bending postures, to extend the length of the exhalation.

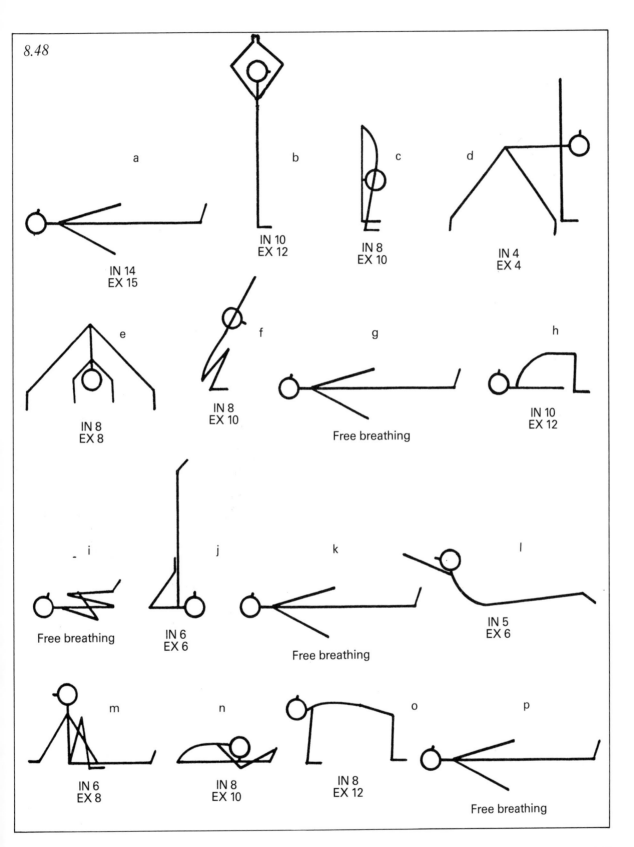

8.48

a

IN 14
EX 15

b

IN 10
EX 12

c

IN 8
EX 10

d

IN 4
EX 4

e

IN 8
EX 8

f

IN 8
EX 10

g

Free breathing

h

IN 10
EX 12

i

Free breathing

j

IN 6
EX 6

k

Free breathing

l

IN 5
EX 6

m

IN 6
EX 8

n

IN 8
EX 10

o

IN 8
EX 12

p

Free breathing

8.49

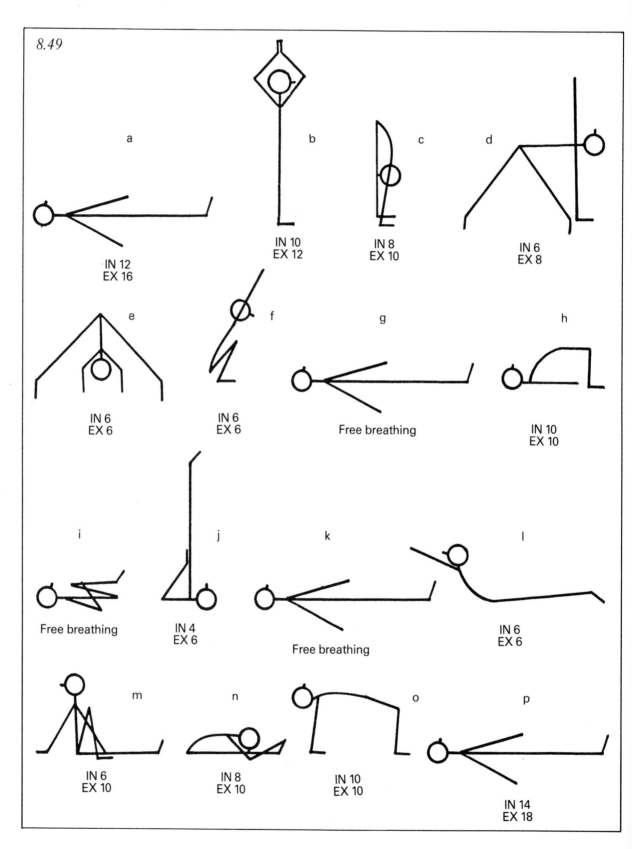

a

b

IN 10
EX 12

c

IN 8
EX 10

d

IN 6
EX 8

IN 12
EX 16

e

IN 6
EX 6

f

IN 6
EX 6

g

Free breathing

h

IN 10
EX 10

i

Free breathing

j

IN 4
EX 6

k

Free breathing

l

IN 6
EX 6

m

IN 6
EX 10

n

IN 8
EX 10

o

IN 10
EX 10

p

IN 14
EX 18

Questions and observations

1 Make notes on your own practice:
  a observing the length and quality of your breath in different postures;
  b comparing the flexibility of your legs and hips in asymmetrical postures.
2 Stand with your back to a wall, so your heels are touching. Inhaling, raise your arms:
  a frontways;
  b sideways;
above your head and observe the movement of your back.
3 Repeat Bhujangasana *(Fig. 8.50)* for four to eight breaths and observe the length of the inhalation on each movement.

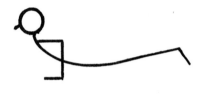

8.50

CHAPTER 9

Pranayama

Pranayama uses your breath to control the finer energy of your body. In this tradition, because we use the breath very precisely in the postures, Pranayama becomes an integrated progression and a natural extension of the practice of asanas which prepare for Pranayama. It is a more refined discipline based upon similar principles to those used in the practice of asanas.

It is unfortunate that an element of mystery has developed around Pranayama, because when it is practised according to the ancient principles it is a safe and beneficial aspect of yoga. However, as with asanas, the personal guidance and instruction of a teacher is essential.

Pranayama is made up of two words, Prana and Ayama. Prana is defined in many different ways in classical texts. It can mean life force, breath, energy, although perhaps the definition of 'finer energy' conveys the most literal meaning. Ayama means to control or to stretch. Thus Pranayama can be defined as the control of finer energy. Prana is the energy which enables life to continue, and when there is no Prana there is no life.

According to an important ancient text, the *Yoga Yagnivalka*, pranic energy flows through the whole body and also extends beyond it *(Fig. 9.1)*. The further Prana extends beyond the body the less effective it becomes, and in mental and physical illness it becomes very dispersed.

Prana, as a finer energy, cannot be directly controlled, but it can be indirectly influenced by the breath and the mind. Yoga has long recognised the profound interrelationship between the breath and the mind. When the mind is agitated, the breath is immediately affected and is disturbed. Conversely, when the breath is slow and controlled, the mind is calm and clear and the pranic energy is more concentrated *(Fig. 9.2)*. Pranayama is a conscious, extremely precise method of making use of these fundamental principles.

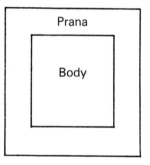

9.1

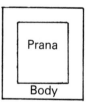

9.2

Posture

It is important that during Pranayama the body is stable. The classical posture for Pranayama is Padmasana *(Fig. 9.3)* and for those who find it comfortable, there are definite advantages in sitting in this posture for Pranayama. Many Indians find Padmasana easy because they have been accustomed to sitting cross-legged from childhood; as a result, their hip, knee and ankle joints have retained their flexibility. For most Westerners, with stiff hip, knee and ankle joints, Padmasana is an unsuitable posture and the quality of the Pranayama will deteriorate because part of the attention is distracted by aching knees and legs — it is essential that the posture should be comfortable.

Ardha Padmasana *(Fig. 9.4)* is a suitable alternative. The posture is fairly easy to master and you should be able to hold it comfortably for ten to twenty minutes with ease. You can place a cushion under your buttocks to help keep the back straight if necessary *(Fig. 9.4a)*.

If these postures are uncomfortable, Siddhasana *(Fig. 9.5)* or, simpler still, Sukhasana *(Fig. 9.6)* are alternatives.

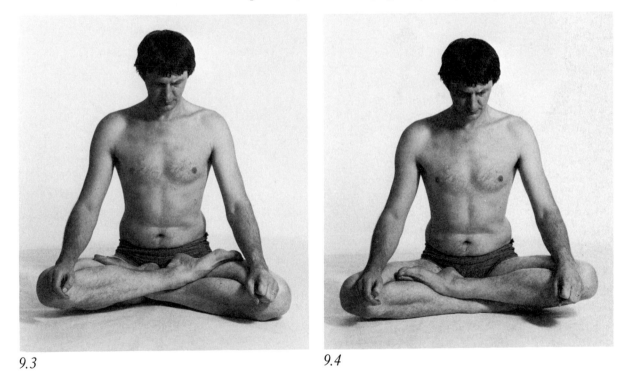

9.3

9.4

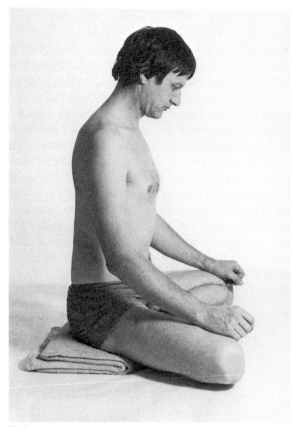

9.4 a

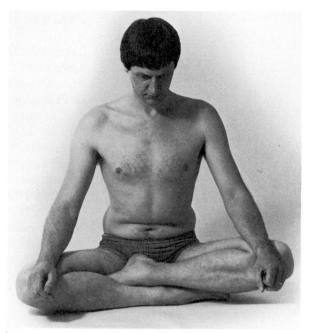

9.5

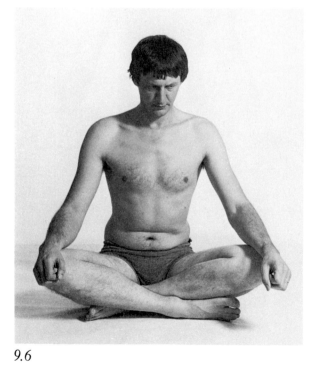

9.6

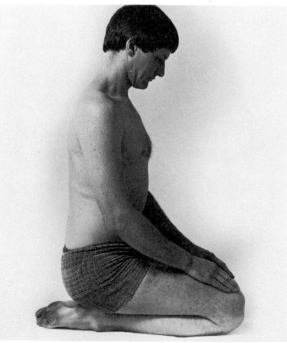

9.7

If you find any cross-legged position difficult, you can sit in Vajrasana *(Fig. 9.7)* for Pranayama although, because your legs are together, it is not as stable as cross-legged postures.

In all cases you should choose a posture you can hold comfortably for the entire length of the Pranayama. It is important that you do not let your back slump after a few minutes and you should use a stool or chair *(Fig. 9.8)* if sitting on the floor is either uncomfortable or results in poor posture. You do not even have to practise Pranayama sitting up; you can practise some simple Pranayamas lying in Savasana.

Why is so much emphasis placed upon having a straight back? There are two main reasons. Firstly, when your back is bent your upper chest is restricted and the upper parts of your lungs cannot be expanded to their full capacity. Secondly, with your back slumped, there is also a restriction of movement in your abdomen, which must be able to expand freely as your diaphragm moves down when your lungs fill. When your back is straight there is freedom of movement and your breathing will be far more effective.

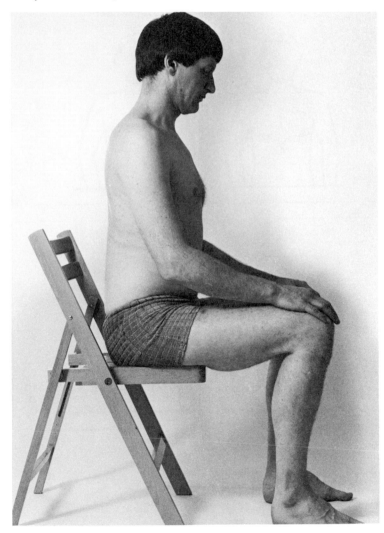

9.8

Methods of breathing

There are two distinctly different ways to breathe. In the first, the inhalation and exhalation begin from the bottom of the lungs and work up to the top *(Fig. 9.9)*. This is quite easy and is suitable not only when you first begin to practise, but also if you have very little movement in your abdomen.

The second method works in the opposite way. The inhalation begins from the top of your lungs and works downwards; the exhalation begins as before from the bottom and works up *(Fig. 9.10)*. One advantage of filling your lungs from the top is that it produces more movement in the upper chest.

Whichever method you use, there should be controlled expanding movement in the ribs, both sideways and forwards, on inhalation, and a contraction during exhalation. For this movement to be controlled properly your mind has to be absorbed in your practice.

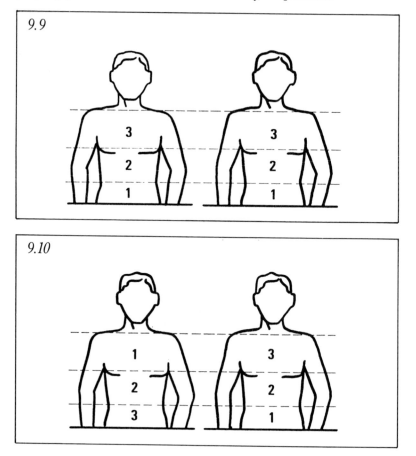

9.9

9.10

Quality of the breath

One of the most important aspects of Pranayama is the quality of the breath. It should be smooth and even and its sound should be constant and controlled. If the sound of your breath begins to vary and becomes harsh or uneven, it is clear that you need to modify your Pranayama.

Division of the breath

In Pranayama there are four parts to each breath:

1 Inhalation (Puraka)
2 Retention of the breath after inhalation (Antah Kumbhaka)
3 Exhalation (Rechaka)
4 Retention after exhalation (Bahya Kumbhaka)

When practising Pranayama the length of the inhalation and exhalation is extended and the breath can be stopped after the inhalation or exhalation or after both.

Pranayamas consist of combinations of these four parts, and the following are examples of some of the permutations:

1 Controlled inhalation and exhalation with no retention.
2 Controlled inhalation and exhalation with retention after inhalation.
3 Controlled inhalation and exhalation with retention after exhalation.
4 Controlled inhalation and exhalation, with retention after inhalation and exhalation.
5 Free inhalation and free exhalation and no retention.
6 Free inhalation with controlled exhalation and no retention.
7 Free inhalation with controlled exhalation and retention after inhalation.
8 Free inhalation with controlled exhalation and retention after exhalation.

(Now you can see why you need a teacher!)

In the following pages, the four parts of the breath — the inhalation, retention of the breath after inhalation, exhalation and retention of the breath after exhalation — will be referred to as IN, H, EX, H, respectively. An inhalation of 6 seconds followed by an exhalation of 12 seconds with retention of 6 seconds would be:

IN (6) : H (0) : EX (12) : H (6)

and would be written as:

6:0:12:6

An inhalation of 8 seconds followed by a retention of 12 seconds after inhalation and an exhalation of 16 seconds with no retention after exhalation would be:

IN (8) : H (12) : EX (16) : H (0)

and would be written as:

8:12:16:0

Counting

Counting the length of the breath

When you are practising Pranayama it is very useful to be able to measure the length of each breath accurately. Counting mentally without external reference is not always very precise and the speed of counting can alter during the practice. To help you attain a greater precision you may find periodic use of a metronome will help you become more precise; set at sixty beats a minute, it provides a reliable reference.

Counting the number of breaths

To help you keep an accurate count of the number of breaths it is helpful to count on the fingers of one hand, using the segments of each finger for each breath. On the first breath place your finger on the bottom segment of your index finger *(Fig. 9.11)*. When you have completed the first breath and are beginning the second inhalation, move your thumb to the second segment *(Fig. 9.12)*. You can continue this process by moving the thumb along from the index finger to the middle finger and so on, giving a total of twelve segments — enough for one round of breaths.

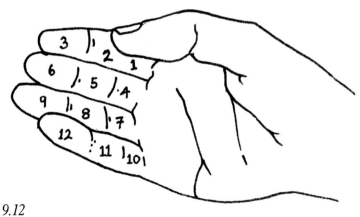

9.11

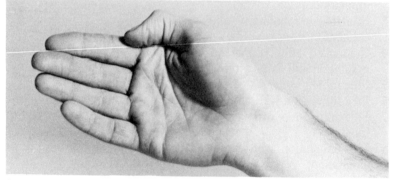

9.12

Ratios

A breathing ratio in Pranayama indicates the relative proportion of one part of the breath to another. Thus a 1:0:2:0 ratio means the exhalation is twice as long as the inhalation, e.g. inhale for 4 seconds, exhale for 8 seconds, or inhale 8 seconds, exhale 16 seconds. The classical Visama-vrtti ratio (1:4:2:0) and Sama-vrtti (1:1:1:1) are well known. A 1:4:2:0 ratio could be 6:24:12:0 or 5:20:10:0, etc. A 1:1:1:1 ratio could be 8:8:8:8 or 10:10:10:10 seconds, etc.

Table 9.1 Examples of different breathing ratios in Pranayama

Ratio	Examples		
1:0:2:0	6:0:12:0	or	10:0:20:0
1:0:1:0	8:0:8:0	or	12:0:12:0
1:1:1:0	9:9:9:0	or	15:15:15:0
1:0:3:0	3:0:9:0	or	6:0:18:0
2:1:2:1	12:6:12:6	or	8:4:8:4

The psychological and physiological effects that different ratios have will vary according to the individual. However, some generalisations can be made, bearing in mind that there will be exceptions to the rule. The use of a longer exhalation, such as 1:0:1½:0, 1:0:2:0 or 1:0:3:0 ratios, often have a relaxing effect. Retention of the breath after the inhalation, such as 1:1:1:0, 1:2:1:0 and 1:4:2:0 ratios, can have a rejuvenating and stimulating effect. Moderate retention of the breath after exhalation, such as 1:0:1:1 and 1:0:2:1 ratios, may tend to calm the mind and make it introverted, while equal ratios, such as 1:1:1:1 or 2:1:2:1, generally have a balancing effect.

The selection of a particular ratio depends upon the psychological and physiological needs of each person, with the psychological needs taking precedence. For example, if you have a very short inhalation you may need to practise retention of the breath after inhalation. However, if you were also tense it would be best to use a ratio with no retention and a longer exhalation so that you could relax. Only then would it be appropriate to work with retention of the breath after inhalation.

The ratio you use during the asanas which precede Pranayama can be selected so that it complements the ratio to be used during the Pranayama. This helps to integrate the two disciplines and Pranayama thus becomes a natural extension of the asanas. For example, if your aim in Pranayama is to work with a longer exhalation, for example 1:0:2:0, this ratio or one similar to it could be used during the principal asanas *(Fig. 9.13)*. You would need to make allowances according to the posture and also to your own breathing capacity.

By working in this way there is both psychological and physiological preparation for Pranayama.

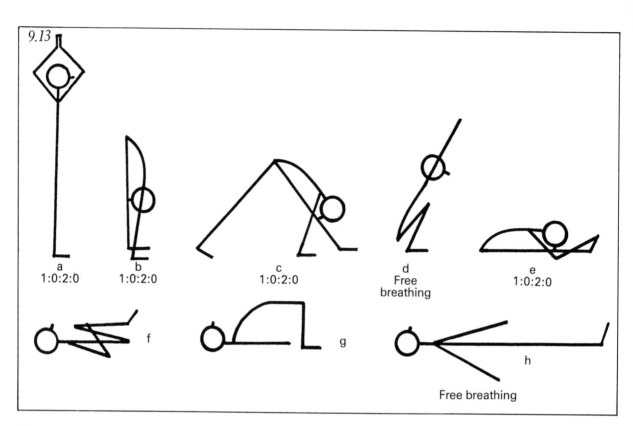

9.13

a
1:0:2:0

b
1:0:2:0

c
1:0:2:0

d
Free
breathing

e
1:0:2:0

f

g

h

Free breathing

Vinyasa in Pranayama

The concept of Vinyasa in Pranayama is precisely the same as in asanas (see Chapter 1). First you need to choose a particular direction or aim, such as attempting 8:16:16:0 in Nadisodhana (see page 154) or 12:12:12:0 in Viloma Ujjayi (see page 153). Then you need to prepare for this by gradually increasing the intensity of the practice in small steps until the goal is reached. The number of breaths in each step is usually between four and twelve and is generally known as a round of breaths, one breath consisting of an inhalation and exhalation. After you have completed the main part of the Pranayama it should be followed by at least one round to taper off. This helps maintain a physiological and psychological balance of:

1 Preparation
2 Goal
3 Descent

(See Fig. 9.14.) The example in Table 9.2 will help to illustrate this idea. Table 9.3 shows a more difficult sequence. The same principle applies to holding after exhalation (Table 9.4) or to an equal ratio (Tables 9.5 and 9.6).

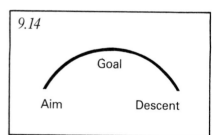

9.14

Goal

Aim

Descent

Table 9.2 Vinyasa in Pranayama

	IN	H	EX	H	Nos of breaths	
Aim	8	16	16	0	12	
Vinyasa						
	8	0	16	0	4	⎫
	8	4	16	0	4	Preparation
	8	8	16	0	4	
	8	12	16	0	4	⎭
	8	16	16	0	12	Main round
	8	0	16	0	6	Relaxing round

Table 9.3 A more difficult Vinyasa in Pranayama

	IN	H	EX	H	Nos of breaths	
Aim	8	16	16	0	12	
Vinyasa						
	8	0	16	0	6	⎱ Preparation
	8	8	16	0	6	⎰
	8	16	16	0	12	Main round
	6	0	12	0	6	Relaxing round

Table 9.4 A Vinyasa leading to holding after exhalation

	IN	H	EX	H	Nos of breaths	
Aim	12	0	12	12	12	
Vinyasa						
	12	0	12	0	4 − 6	⎫
	12	0	12	4	4 − 6	Preparation
	12	0	12	8	4 − 6	⎭
	12	0	12	12	12	Main round
	8	0	10	0	6	Relaxing round

Table 9.5 Vinyasa leading to an equal ratio

	IN	H	EX	H	Nos of breaths	
Aim	8	8	8	8	12	
Vinyasa						
	8	0	8	0	4	⎫
	8	8	8	0	6	Preparation
	8	0	8	8	6	⎭
	8	8	8	8	12	Main round
	6	0	6	0	6	Relaxing round

Table 9.6 Vinyasa leading to equal breaths and equal retentions

	IN	H	EX	H	Nos of breaths
Aim	10	5	10	5	12
Vinyasa					
	10	0	10	0	6 } Preparation
	10	5	10	0	6 }
	10	5	10	0	12 Main round
	8	0	8	0	6 Relaxing round

At first the initial increase in the length of each breath or retention between each step needs to be small — say 2 to 4 seconds. As you become more proficient these steps can be lengthened to between 6 and 12 seconds.

Combinations of Pranayamas

You can include more than one type of Pranayama in one practice. Simpler Pranayama with easy ratios can be used as preparation for the main part of the practice. If, for example, your aim was 12:12:12:0 in Nadisodhana (see page 154) then you could use Anuloma Ujjayi (see page 153) 12:0:24:0 × 12 breaths as preparation. Nadisodhana could be followed by Ujjayi (see page 152) with a shorter ratio to act as a counter-balance (see Table 9.7). Another example could be as in Table 9.8, where Anuloma Ujjayi and Viloma Ujjayi act as preparation for Nadisodhana. Sitali (see page 155) is also a good preparation at the beginning of a Pranayama.

There are many other combinations. The type of Pranayama and the ratio you choose must be related to the main aim of the Pranayama and to your individual needs.

Table 9.7 An example of a combination of Pranayamas

	IN	H	EX	H	Nos of breaths
Anuloma Ujjayi	12	0	24	0	6 }
Nadisodhana	12	6	12	0	6 } Preparation
	12	8	12	0	6 }
	12	12	12	0	12 Main round
Ujjayi	6	0	12	0	4 Relaxing round

Table 9.8 Another combination of Pranayamas

	IN	H	EX	H	Nos	of breaths
Anuloma Ujjayi	6	0	12	0	6	Preparation
Viloma Ujjayi	12	0	12	0	6	
Nadisodhana	12	0	12	0	12	Main round
Ujjayi	Free breathing				6	Relaxing round

Advantages of Vinyasa

1 Many students who find it enjoyable and beneficial to practise asanas often find Pranayama tedious and boring. But, by using the principle of Vinyasa, there is more direction for the mind and this improves concentration. You can also use Vinyasa to improve the length of breath and retention.

2 Gradually increasing the intensity of the Pranayama results in a better mental and physical preparation, and this in turn often improves your Pranayama. For example, if you were asked to practise retention after inhalation without preparation you might be able to do 4:8:8:0, but by using a Vinyasa you could extend the retention to longer periods. It is lack of *mental* preparation which sometimes prevents you reaching your full capacity.

3 By using Vinyasa you avoid launching into something too strenuous too soon. By gradually building up to your main goal you are able to observe and control the accumulative effect of your Pranayama, changing and modifying its form when necessary as you go along.

4 Your breathing capacity will vary from day to day and is influenced by many different factors — time of year, weather, emotions, fatigue, etc. Vinyasa helps you become sensitive to these changes and to modify the Pranayama accordingly.

Controlling the breath

There are several techniques for controlling the flow of breath.

Throat control

One of the simplest ways of getting a finer control of the breath is to constrict your throat slightly while still breathing through your nostrils. This has two effects.

1 It gives you greater control of the breath, making it longer and more even.

2 The constriction makes your breath audible and so acts as a useful indication of its quality. If the control is correct the sound will be even and gentle. If the *constriction* is too strong the sound will be harsh and too loud.

This type of breathing, where the inhalation and exhalation are controlled at the throat, is called Ujjayi.

Finger control

The technique of using your fingers to regulate your breath, on the inhalation or exhalation or both, gives you a great deal more control over your breath. The index and middle fingers are bent onto the palm and generally the third finger and the thumb of your right hand are placed on the left and right sides of the nose respectively, just below where the bone finishes *(Fig. 9.15)* — vice versa for the left hand. The inhalation or exhalation is controlled by closing one nostril with either your finger or thumb and applying a small amount of pressure on the other nostril with the other finger. Avoid pushing the nostrils too hard or turning your head.

The advantages of controlling your breath with the fingers is that the length of the breath can be increased and the control itself becomes more refined and sensitive. If in Ujjayi the length of your breath is 8 seconds on inhalation and 12 on exhalation, with finger control you could extend this to an inhalation of 12 seconds and an exhalation of 16 seconds.

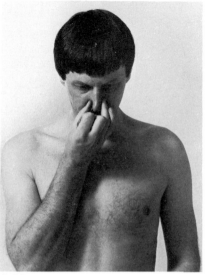

9.15

Different Pranayamas

It is important to realise that different Pranayamas have different effects upon different people. However, we can make some generalisations.

Pranayamas can be divided into four groups:

1 Pranayama with throat control only.
2 Pranayama with throat and finger control.
3 Pranayama with finger control only.
4 Pranayama with inhalation through mouth.

Pranayama with throat control only

Ujjayi
IN throat
EX throat
Ujjayi Pranayama is one of the simplest types of Pranayama. As there is no control of the breath with the fingers, full attention can be given to the controlled inhalation and exhalation through the throat. You may find it useful to start with Ujjayi when first beginning to practise Pranayama under the supervision of your teacher.

Pranayama with throat and finger control

Some Pranayamas are a combination of Ujjayi and controlling the breath with the fingers. They are Anuloma Ujjayi, Viloma Ujjayi and Pratiloma Ujjayi.

Anuloma Ujjayi
IN throat
EX left nostril
IN throat
EX right nostril

In Anuloma Ujjayi you inhale through both nostrils, with the breath controlled at the throat, and you exhale, using finger control, through alternate nostrils.

This Pranayama is often useful when first learning to control the breath with your fingers because it is easier for you to exhale than to inhale through a nostril using finger control, since often one or both nostrils are partially blocked and need to be cleansed. By controlling the exhalation with your fingers it is possible to have more control over the length of your exhalation and this makes it suitable to be used with ratios where the exhalation is longer, e.g. 1:0:2:0 or 1:0:3:0. It can also be used with retention after the inhalation or exhalation, depending on your individual needs.

Viloma Ujjayi
IN right nostril
EX throat
IN left nostril
EX throat

Viloma Ujjayi is the opposite technique of Anuloma Ujjayi. In this Pranayama you inhale through one nostril, using finger control, and exhale through both nostrils, with your breath controlled at the throat. This gives you more control over the inhalation and is useful when you need to extend the length of your inhalation. It can also be used as a preparation for Pratiloma Ujjayi and Nadisodhana.

Pratiloma Ujjayi
IN throat
EX left nostril
IN left nostril
EX throat
IN throat
EX right nostril
IN right nostril
EX throat

Pratiloma Ujjayi is a combination of Ujjayi, Anuloma Ujjayi and Viloma Ujjayi, and you can use it for a number of reasons.

If during your practice of simpler Pranayama you cannot concentrate, Pratiloma, because it is more complex and intricate, may help you keep your attention centred. It is most suited to be used with a Samana, or equal ratio, e.g. 1:1:1:1 or 2:1:2:1.

Pranayamas with finger control only

Nadisodhana
IN right nostril
EX left nostril
IN left nostril
EX right nostril
In Nadisodhana you control your breath with your fingers, both on the inhalation and exhalation. By varying the degree of pressure used with the finger or thumb on the inhalation or exhalation, your breath can be altered in a variety of ways. This makes it very adaptable and allows you to use many different types of ratio such as 1:0:1:0, 1:0:2:0, 1:1:1:0, 1:2:2:2 and 1:0:2:1, 2:1:2:1.

Suryabhedana and Candrabhedana
In Suryabhedana:
IN right nostril
EX left nostril
IN right nostril
EX left nostril
and Candrabhedana:
IN left nostril
EX right nostril
IN left nostril
EX right nostril
The inhalation is constant through one nostril and the exhalation is constant through the opposite nostril. These Pranayamas are useful as preparation for Nadisodhana when one nostril is blocked with mucus. You can often remove the blockage by inhaling through the clear nostril and exhaling through the blocked nostril. Retention of the breath after inhalation will often aid this process.

Bhastrika
IN right nostril
EX left nostril
IN left nostril
EX right nostril
This is the same technique as that used in Nadisodhana but the inhalation and exhalation are very fast. You should not attempt this Pranayama until you have achieved good control of your breath in Nadisodhana.

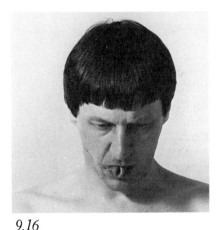

9.16

Pranayama with inhalation through the mouth

Sitali

1 IN tongue
   EX throat
2 IN tongue
   EX left nostril
   IN tongue
   EX right nostril

In Sitali *(Fig. 9.16)* the lips are formed into a circle and the tip of the tongue, which is curled upwards at the sides, protrudes half an inch from the lips.

You inhale through your mouth as you raise your head. The exhalation is either controlled through the throat or with the fingers as your head is lowered.

Practising Pranayama

All these examples show that there are many factors which need to be considered when practising Pranayama. Considerable training and experience are required to select the most appropriate Pranayamas and ratios for each individual. Direct and constant supervision are required to practise Pranayama correctly.

Questions and observations

1 Observe your breath during a simple asana practice and choose a ratio and type of Pranayama which will help improve control of either the inhalation or exhalation.
2 Practise and then compare the following ratios in
   a Anuloma Ujjayi
   b Ujjayi
   1:0:1:0
   1:0:2:0
   1:1:2:0
   1:0:1:1
3 Prepare a simple Vinyasa using two types of Pranayama as preparation for Nadisodhana, using one of the following ratios in Nadisodhana.
   a $1:\frac{1}{2}:1:0$
   b $1:0:1:\frac{1}{2}$
   c $1:\frac{1}{2}:1:\frac{1}{2}$

CHAPTER 10

Planning a Practice

The basis of this tradition is that the practice of Asanas and Pranayama is adapted to the individual; what is right for you is not going to be suitable for someone else. The sequence of postures, their counter-poses, variations, modifications, etc., need to be selected to suit your own needs and your practice needs to be revised as you yourself change and progress.

General comments

The following general notes need to be kept in mind.

Need for a teacher

You should not practise asanas and Pranayama without the direct and constant supervision of a competent teacher who has himself studied directly from a teacher who comes from an authentic and living tradition.

Medical problems

If you have a particular medical problem such as a slipped disc, sciatica, epilepsy, high or low blood pressure or heart disease, you must take great care with your practice and it is especially important that you should be supervised by your teacher.

Mental attitude

There should be no competition in the practice of yoga, either with yourself or with other people. The degree to which you can move into a posture, or the length of time the breath can be held in Pranayama, are not the main criteria for good practice. It is your mental attitude, the depth of concentration and your involvement and one-pointedness in your practice which are most important. As you practise, focus your attention more and more so that your concentration becomes deeper, and one asana flows into the next.

Preparation

There are several ways you can help prepare yourself for your practice. If you do your practice first thing in the morning, you may find it helpful to take a shower or a cool bath as this helps relax some of the morning stiffness. If you are practising late in the day, after you have been busy, it may help you to allow a short period of quietness before starting. Do not practise immediately after a meal but allow three or four hours to elapse so that digestion can occur.

Vinyasa

Before you start it is a good idea to plan the sequence of your practice, either mentally or by jotting down on a piece of paper the precise structure of the postures and/or type of Pranayama, etc. This will help, first of all, to keep your attention in the practice and, secondly, to avoid continually repeating the most familiar asanas. The practice itself should be creative, alive and alert, not dull and routine. If your attention is not completely involved with your practice and if your mind is somewhere else, the result will be far less effective. Once you have been taught and understand the basic principles of Vinyasa in asanas and Pranayama, you can experiment under guidance, trying different sequences and different ratios, etc.

Sthira and Sukha

The *Yoga Sutras of Patanjali* say there should be two qualities present in the practice of asanas: one is Sthira and the other Sukha. Sthira means stability, firmness, and to be in the present: Sukha means being at ease, and the elimination of tension. So when you are in a particular asana there should be no strain, no tension. The ability to recognise when you are working within your capacity without strain is an important part of the practice of asanas and Pranayama. If you work with too much force — mentally or physically — without accepting your limitations, then your practice can have harmful psychological and physiological effects.

Regularity

Regularity is another very important point to remember in your practice. If possible you should practise every day, even if it is only for a short time. This is much better than practising once a week for two hours. Try to practise each day at the same time, preferably in the morning and in the same place.

Breathing

Remember that all movements in the postures should be synchronised with the breath.

157

Planning

The previous chapters have each outlined the different principles of practising asanas and Pranayama. Each of these has a profound effect and needs to be carefully considered. By varying some or all of these principles you can produce a great many permutations with only one Vinyasa. To refresh your memory the points you need to remember are as follows:

1 Vinyasa — the order of asanas, from preparation to the main goal and descent.
2 Counter-pose.
3 Use of breath, i.e. breathing ratios and the time spent in each asana.
4 Dynamic or static use of asanas.
5 Variation of asanas.
6 Modification of asanas.

When planning a practice decide on the main goal, such as holding Pascimatanasana for eighteen breaths in a particular breathing ratio, e.g. 6:0:12:6, or holding Sarvangasana for twelve breaths, using different variations.

Take into account your particular mental and physical condition and adapt your practice accordingly. At first you will need the help of your teacher to do this.

Plan the preparation and descent and also relate this to the Pranayama which may follow.

The following examples will help to illustrate how one simple practice can be varied a great deal by changing any of these six principles. The basic Vinyasa is shown in Fig. 10.1, but this can be varied as follows:

1 Varying the number of breaths *(Figs. 10.2 and 10.3)*.

2 Varying the breathing ratio in the principal postures *(Figs. 10.4 and 10.5)*.

3 Varying the modification *(Figs. 10.6 and 10.7)*.

4 Varying the dynamic and static use of postures *(Figs 10.8 and 10.9)*.

5 Varying the counter-poses *(Figs. 10.10 and 10.11)*.

6 Changing the variations *(Figs. 10.12 and 10.13)*.

On pages 172—227 examples of how the principles in the previous chapters are applied. They include a simple Vinyasa, two moderate Vinyasas and one vigorous Vinyasa.

10.1

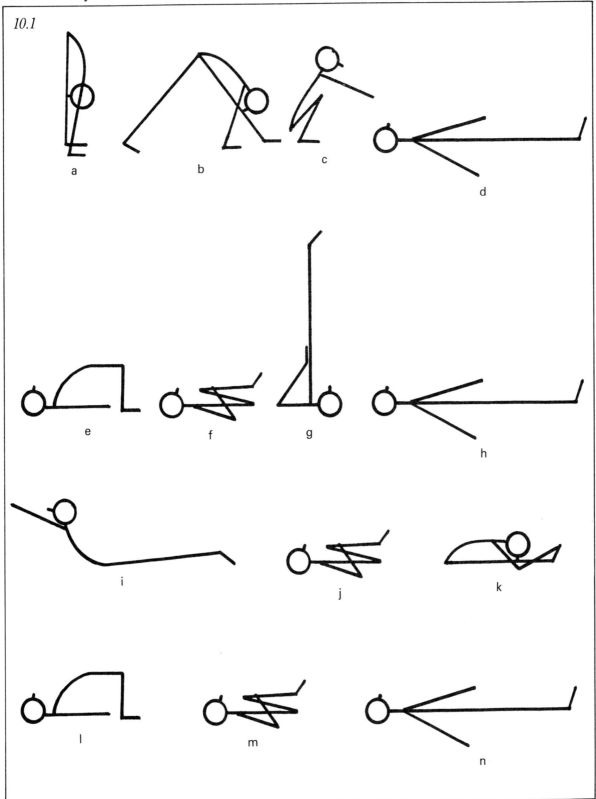

10.2

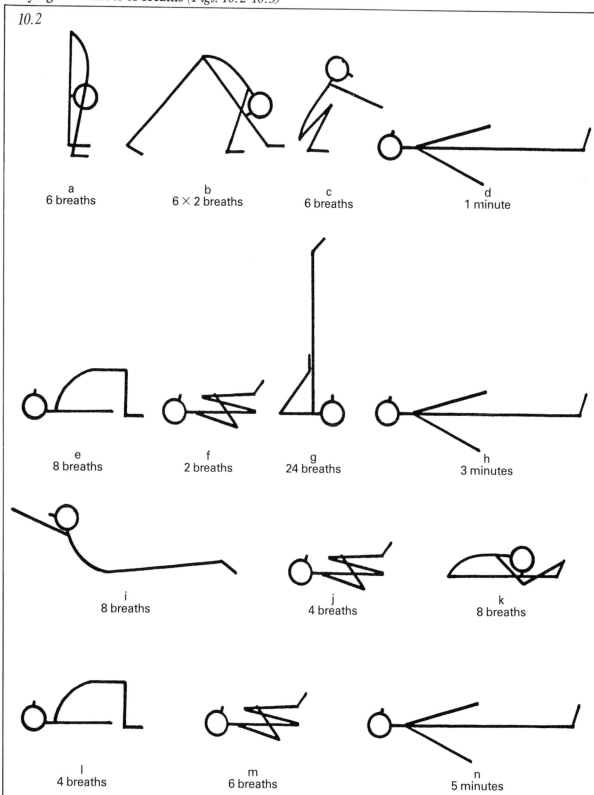

a
6 breaths

b
6 × 2 breaths

c
6 breaths

d
1 minute

e
8 breaths

f
2 breaths

g
24 breaths

h
3 minutes

i
8 breaths

j
4 breaths

k
8 breaths

l
4 breaths

m
6 breaths

n
5 minutes

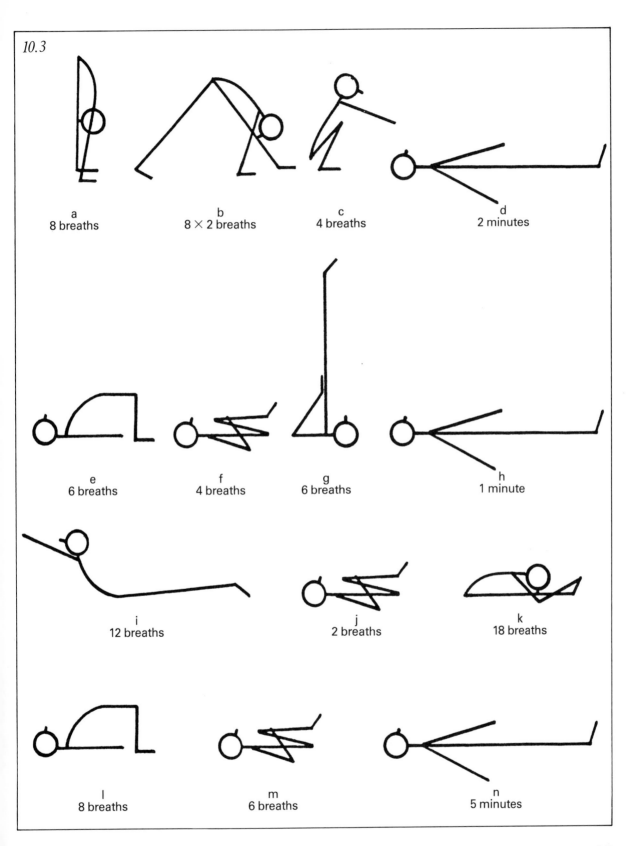

10.3

a
8 breaths

b
8 × 2 breaths

c
4 breaths

d
2 minutes

e
6 breaths

f
4 breaths

g
6 breaths

h
1 minute

i
12 breaths

j
2 breaths

k
18 breaths

l
8 breaths

m
6 breaths

n
5 minutes

10.4

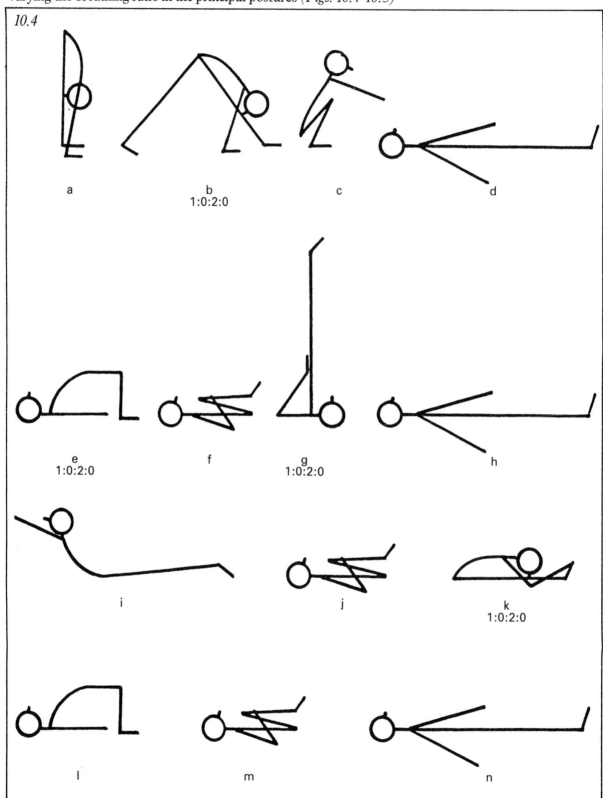

a

b
1:0:2:0

c

d

e
1:0:2:0

f

g
1:0:2:0

h

i

j

k
1:0:2:0

l

m

n

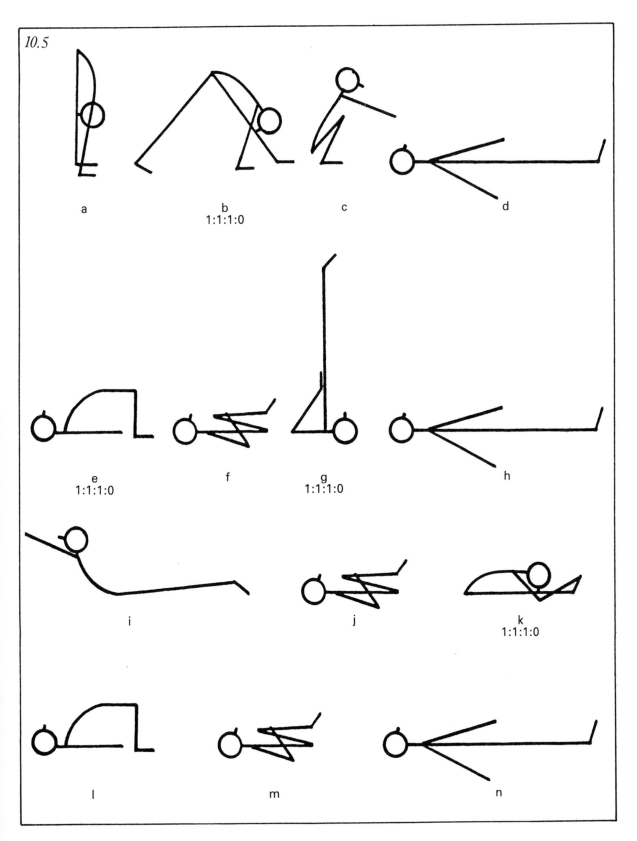

a

b
1:1:1:0

c

d

e
1:1:1:0

f

g
1:1:1:0

h

i

j

k
1:1:1:0

l

m

n

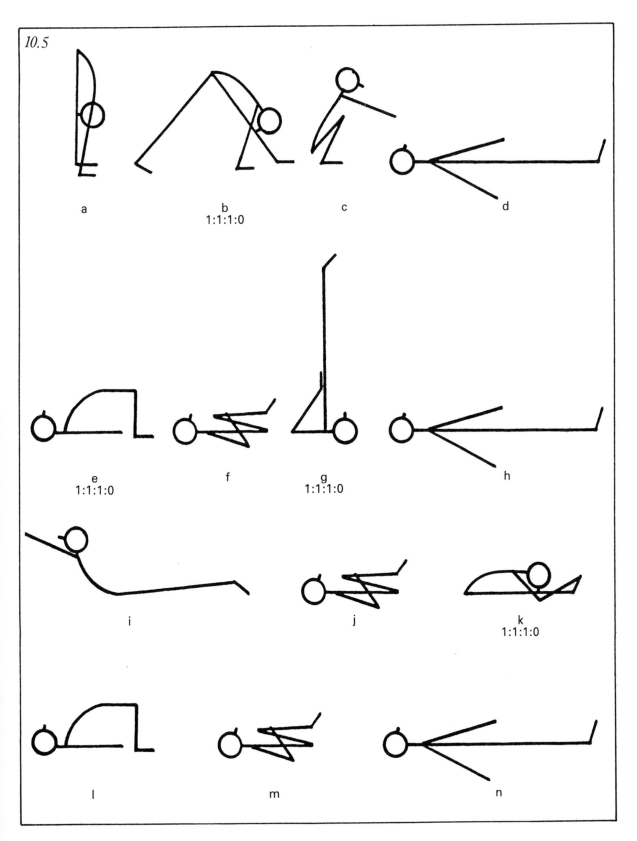

10.6

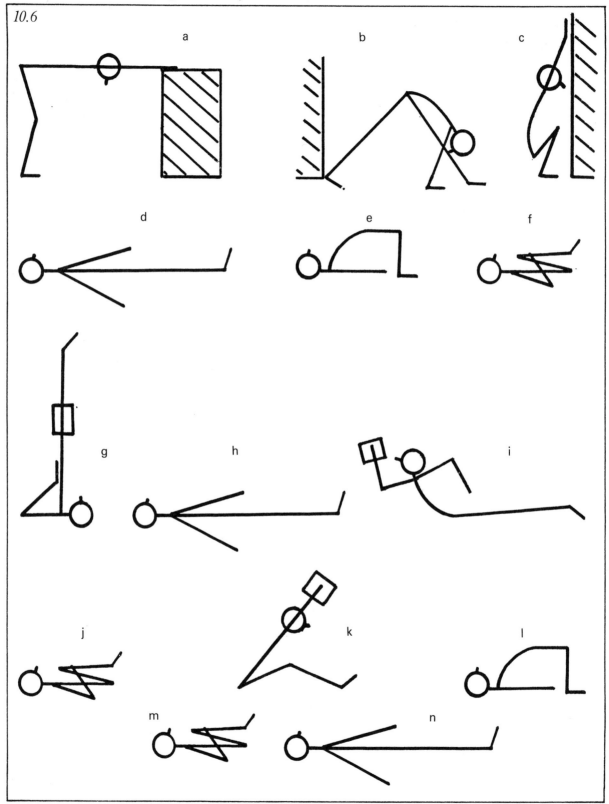

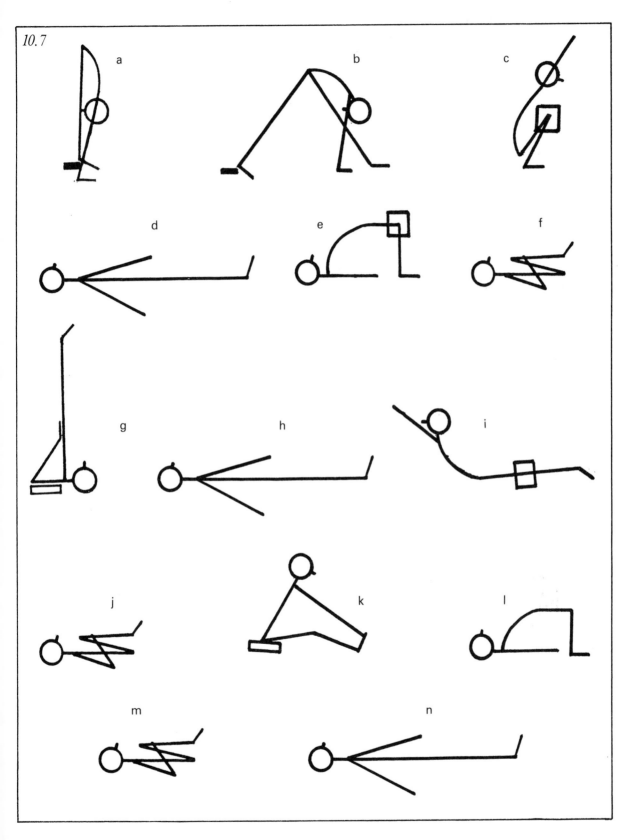

10.8

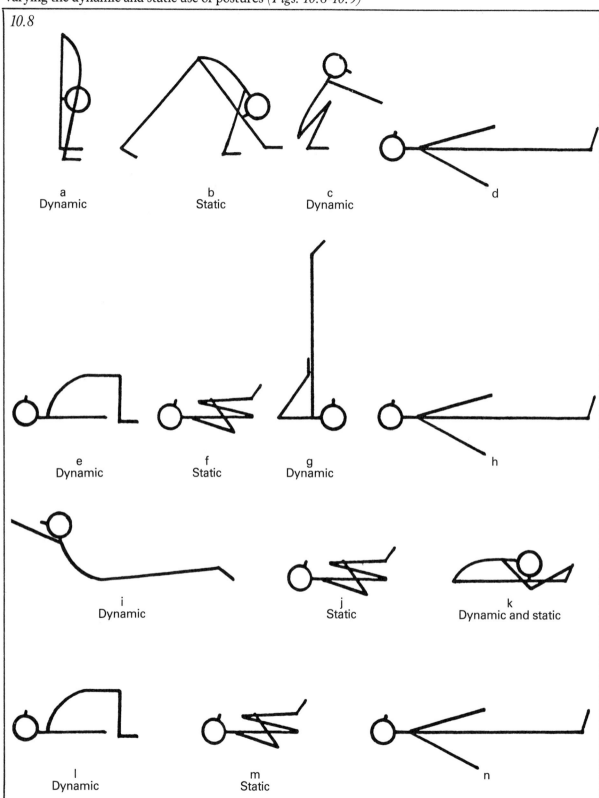

a
Dynamic

b
Static

c
Dynamic

d

e
Dynamic

f
Static

g
Dynamic

h

i
Dynamic

j
Static

k
Dynamic and static

l
Dynamic

m
Static

n

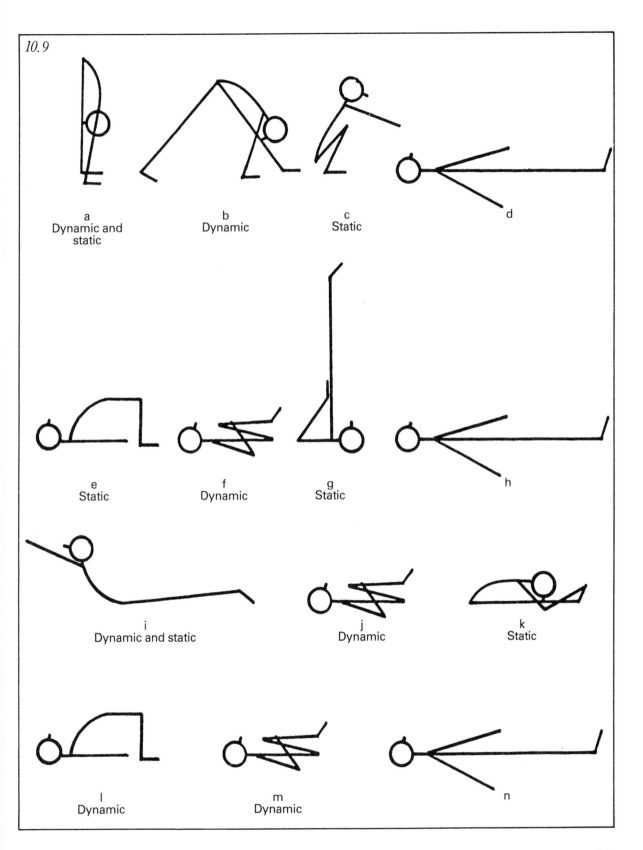

10.9

a
Dynamic and
static

b
Dynamic

c
Static

d

e
Static

f
Dynamic

g
Static

h

i
Dynamic and static

j
Dynamic

k
Static

l
Dynamic

m
Dynamic

n

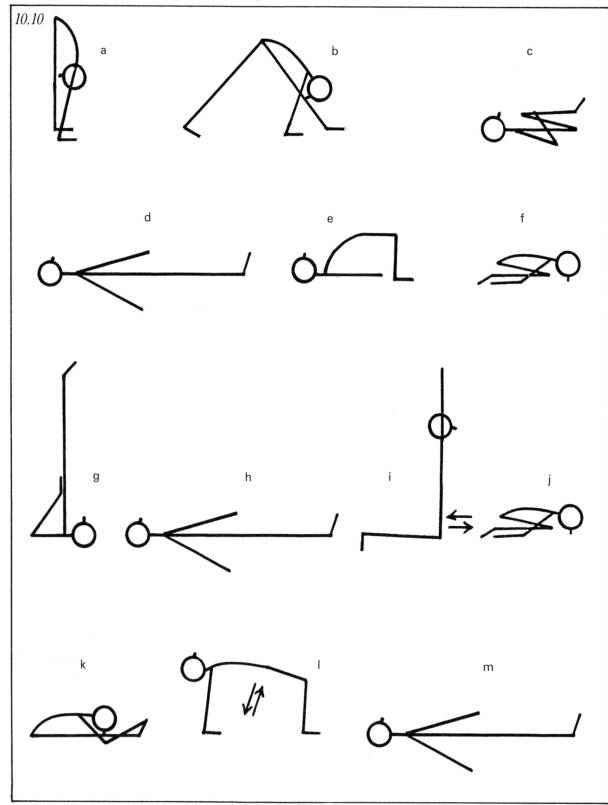

10.10

a

b

c

d

e

f

g

h

i

j

k

l

m

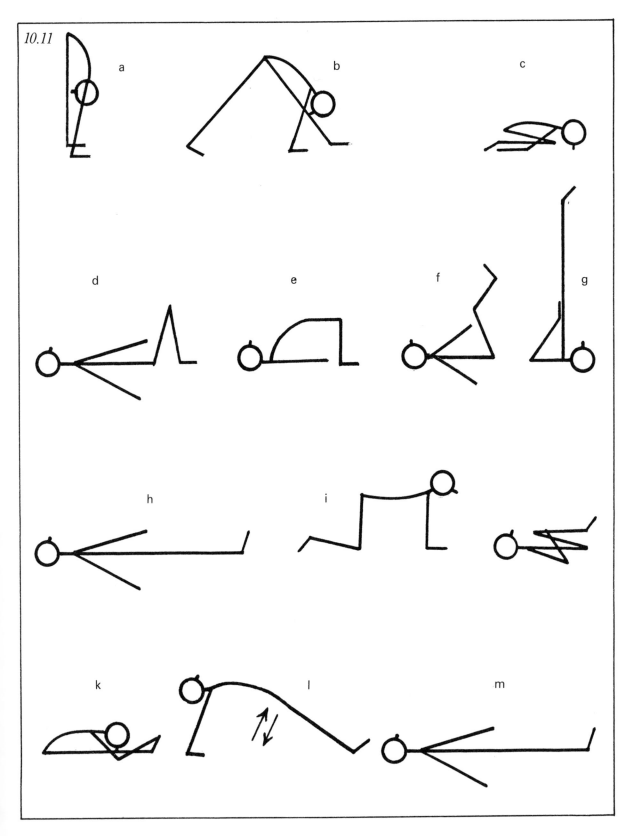

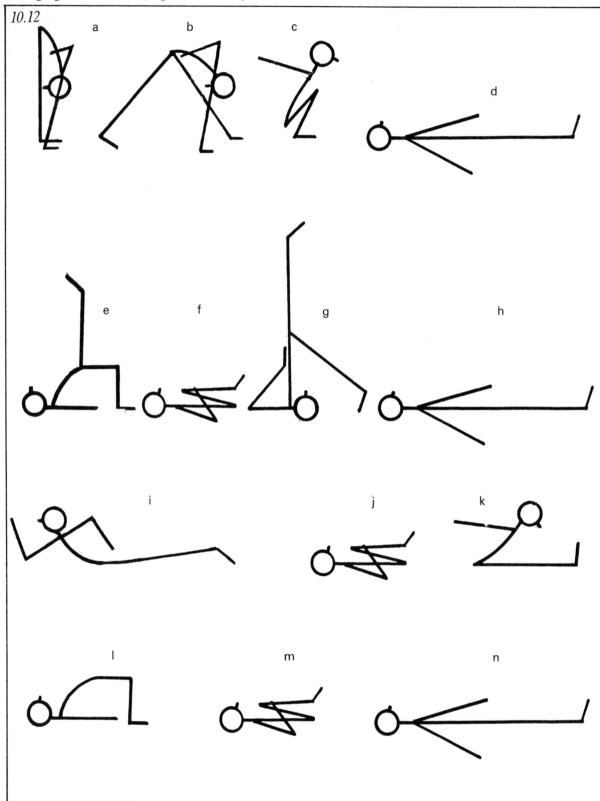

10.12

a b c d e f g h i j k l m n

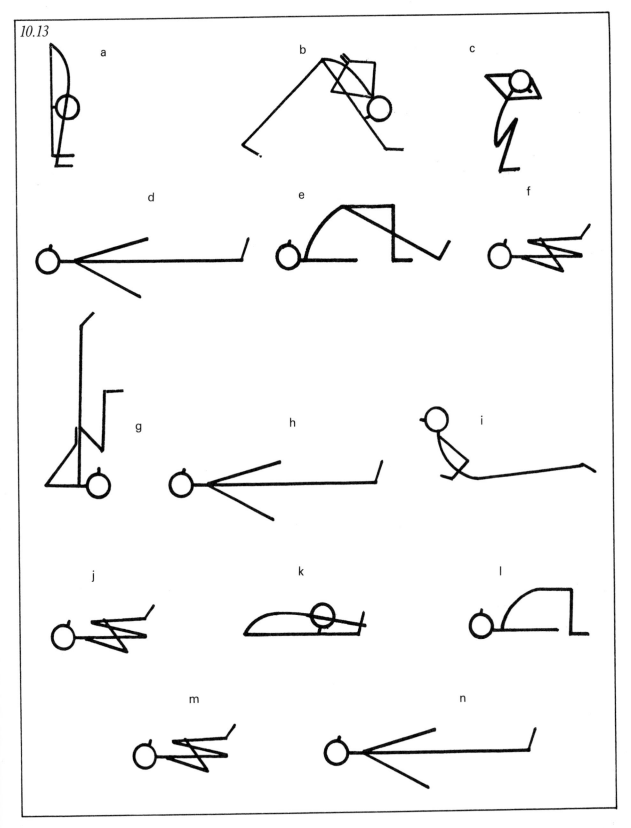

Example 1 — A Vinyasa for Ardha Uttanasana

Explanatory notes

The first example is a very simple Vinyasa and is not at all strenuous. The main posture is Ardha Uttanasana *(Fig. 10.14)* which has been modified in two ways to make it easier. First, by placing your hands on a table-top, your back does not have to support the weight of your trunk and arms. Second, your legs can be bent, allowing more movement in your back. Your arms can also be bent to allow more freedom of movement in the upper back, shoulders and neck.

The main posture comes towards the end of the Vinyasa *(Fig. 10.15)*. The first postures are lying postures (a, b and c), followed by kneeling postures (d and e), which lead to and prepare for the standing asanas (f and g). The Vinyasa begins with slow breathing in Savasana (a), which is followed by Supta Ekapada Prasrta Padasana (b); this stretches the legs and also works the lower back. This is followed by Supta Prasrta Padasana (c), with the same movement using both legs; your legs are bent first onto the chest and then raised and lowered. This variation is much easier than when your legs are raised up directly from the lying position. In Cakravakasana (d) your spine is moved one way and the other into concave and convex positions. Vajrasana (e) prepares your spine for the forward-bending movement in Ardha Uttanasana. The posture is used dynamically, and is made easier by sweeping your arms behind your back on the downward movement. Used statically, it acts as a counter-pose for Cakravakasana.

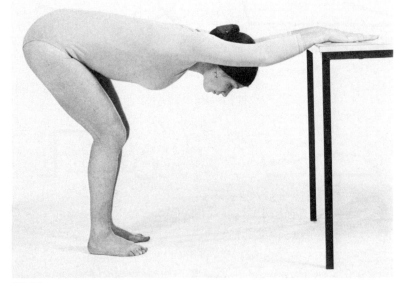

10.14

The standing sequence of postures begins with Tadasana (f). This posture can be practised with your back to a wall, which both acts as a reference point and helps to ensure that your back does not arch too much as your arms are raised. Having thoroughly prepared the main postures, Ardha Uttanasana can now be practised, this being followed by the counter-pose Apanasana (h) and a rest of five minutes in Savasana (i). The sequence of Asanas is followed by a few minutes of slow breathing in Savasana (j) and completed by a period of relaxation in Savasana (k).

A Vinyasa of this type is often suitable for people who are just starting to practise asanas or who are restarting their practice after illness.

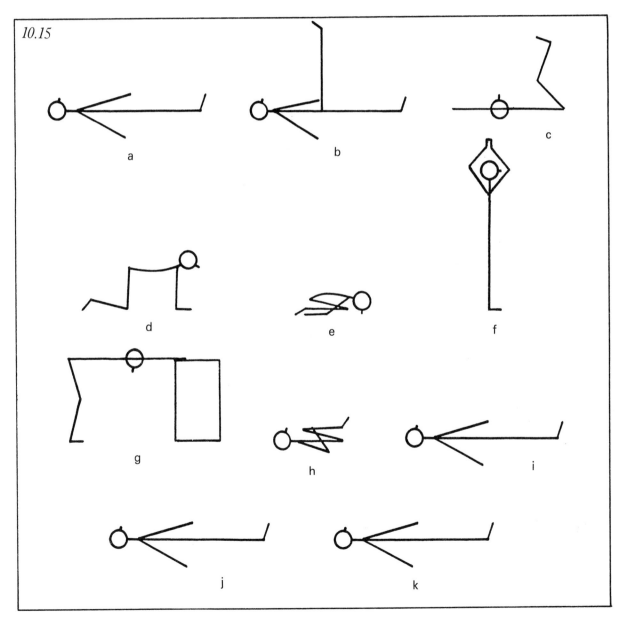

10.15

a

b

c

d

e

f

g

h

i

j

k

(a) Savasana — corpse pose

It is very important for you to approach your practice with the right mental attitude. Do not rush straight into the asanas, but gradually bring your mind towards your practice.

1 Lie down on your back on a thick blanket or rug on the floor. Your body should be straight, with the head down slightly, your hands a few inches away from your body with the palms turned upwards *(Fig. 10.16)*. Keep your eyes closed.

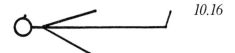

10.16

2 For a few minutes simply observe your body lying on the floor.
3 As your attention becomes more centred, begin to observe your breath on the inhalation and exhalation, noting its quality and length. It should be even from beginning to end. The quality of your breath is determined to a great extent by the quality of your concentration, so give your full attention to each breath.
4 Gradually extend the length of your breath, inhaling through your nose and controlling the breath at the throat, so it gives a soft, even sound.
5 Start your inhalation from the top of your chest, gradually expanding downwards. Observe the forward and sideways movement of your ribs and control the expansion of your abdomen as the diaphragm moves downwards.
6 Start the exhalation by slightly contracting your abdomen, then allow your lower ribs to contract and finally allow the upper chest to contract.
7 Continue until your mind is in tune with your body.

There are a number of variations and modifications to this posture. Try some of those in Fig. 10.17 and compare the effects.

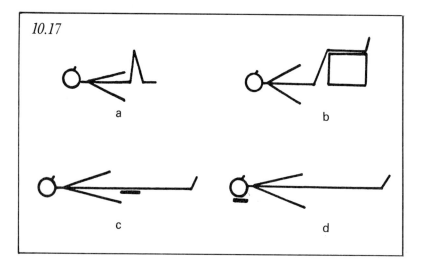

10.17

a

b

c

d

(b) Ekapada Urdhva Prasrta Padasana (modified) — one-leg-upward stretched-leg pose

10.18

1 Lie on your back with your arms at your side and your legs straight (a). Inhale.

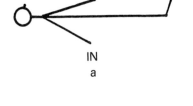

IN
a

2 Exhaling, bend your right leg onto your chest (b), making sure the movement is synchronised with your breath.

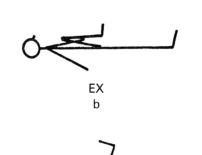

EX
b

3 Inhaling, straighten your right leg up and raise both your arms, taking them over your head and onto the floor (c).

IN
c

4 Exhaling, lower your right leg back onto your chest and bring your arms back (d).

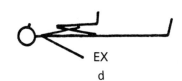

EX
d

Repeat for four breaths and then change to your left leg. Remember to synchronise each movement with your breathing.

If you find it is difficult to keep your arms straight as they go over your head, bend your elbows.

Observe the changes in your back, hips and muscles in the back of your legs between the raising of each leg.

(c) Urdhva Prasrta Padasana (modified) — upward stretched-leg pose

1 Lie on your back with your arms at your side and your legs straight (a). Inhale.

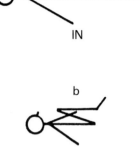

a

IN

2 Exhaling, bend both your legs onto your chest (b).

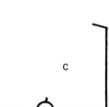

b

EX

3 Inhaling, straighten both your legs up in the air as you take your arms over your head (c).

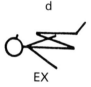

c

IN

4 Exhaling, lower your legs back onto your chest, bring your arms back (d).

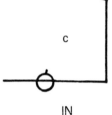

d

EX

Repeat for six breaths.

Do not allow your head to come up as your legs are raised and lowered.

Compare this posture with the previous one.

(d) Cakravakasana (modified) — bird pose

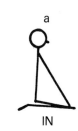

a

IN

1 Sit on your heels, with your legs together (a). Inhale.

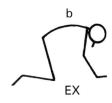

b

EX

2 Exhaling, bend forward and place your hands on the floor 12—18 inches in front of your knees (b).

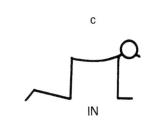

c

IN

3 Inhaling, lift your buttocks up off your heels until your legs are vertical to the floor (c). Your arms and legs should be parallel as your back bends, and as your chest expands and your head is raised.

d

EX

4 Exhaling, bend your elbows and move your body backwards, arching your back and lowering your head (d).

Repeat for six breaths.
   Avoid hunching your shoulders.

(e) Vajrasana — spine pose

1 Sit on your heels with your hands on your knees (a).

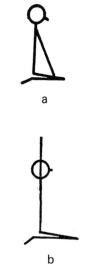

a

2 Inhaling, raise your arms above your head, elbows slightly bent (b).

b

3 Exhaling, bend forward, sweeping your arms to your side. Lower your forehead onto the floor and place your hands by your feet (c).

c

Stay for six breaths, relaxing into the posture.

    This posture is a counter-pose to the previous postures. If it is not comfortable you can use Apanasana (page 183) instead.

(f) Tadasana — palm tree pose

10.22

1 Stand in Samasthiti with your body straight, with your back towards a wall and your heels 2 inches or so away from the bottom of the wall (a).

a

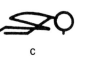

2 Inhaling, slowly raise your arms forwards and above your head (b). Observe the movement in your lower back and the effect of the movement in your upper back, shoulders and neck.

b

3 Exhaling, lower your arms (c).

Repeat for eight breaths.
   If, because of stiffness in your back or shoulders, the movement of
your arms is restricted, bend your elbows *(Fig. 10.23)*.
   Observe the effect that the movement of your arms has on the upper
and lower parts of your back.

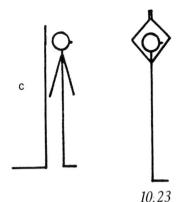

c

10.23

(g) Ardha Uttanasana — half-forward stretched pose

10.24

1 Stand in Samasthiti 3 feet in front of a table with your feet 6—9
   inches apart (a).

a

2 Inhaling, raise your arms above your head, bending your arms
   slightly (b).

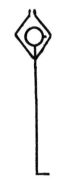

b
IN

3 Exhaling, bend forward, keeping your arms back and your chest
   open. Bend your knees slightly, placing your hands on the top of the
   table (c). Keep your arms bent.

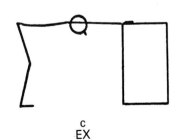

c
EX

179

4 Inhaling, look up and open your chest (d).

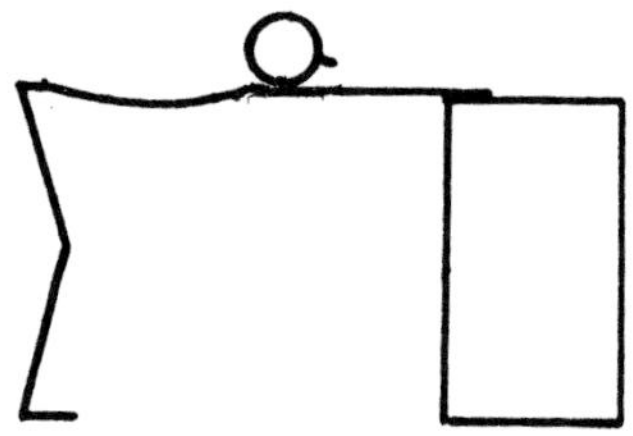

d
IN

5 Exhaling, lower your head (e).

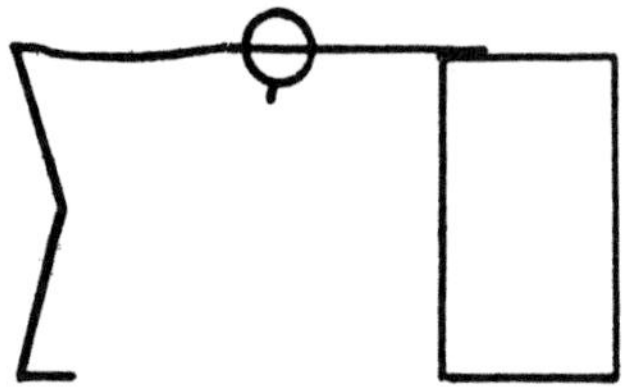

e
EX

6 Repeat for eight breaths.

7 Inhaling, come up from the posture, raising your arms first (f).

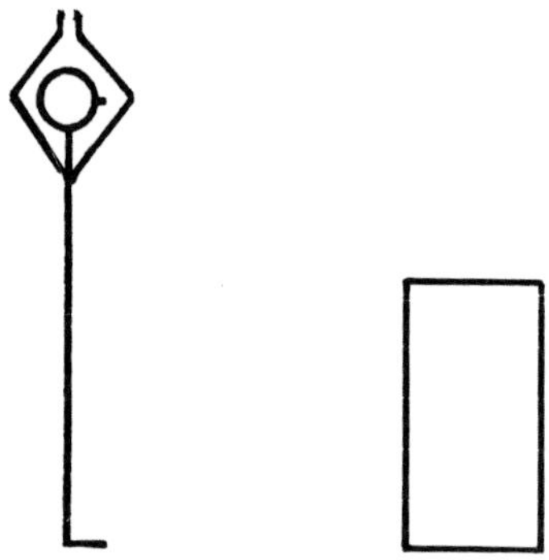

f
IN

8 Exhaling, lower your arms (g).

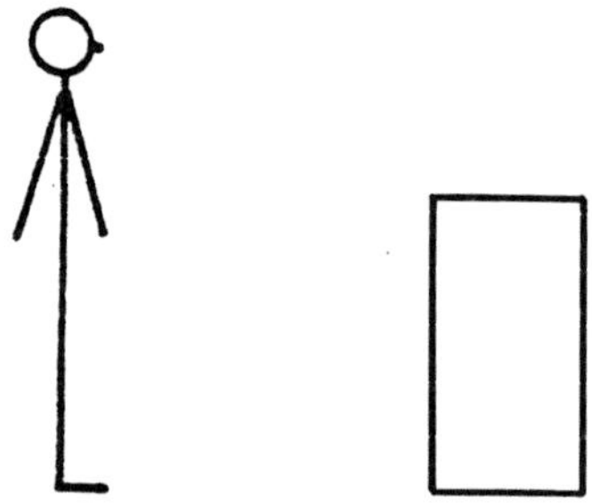

g
EX

Try working with your legs straight in this posture, and compare it with when your legs are bent.

(h) Apanasana (counter-pose) — lower abdomen pose

10.25

1 Lying on your back, inhale (a).

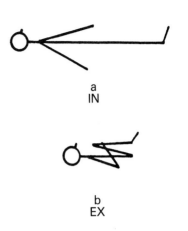

a
IN

2 Exhaling, bend your knees onto your abdomen and place your hands on your knees (b).

Hold for six breaths.

b
EX

(i) Savasana — corpse pose

Inhale and carefully straighten your legs onto the floor. Place your hands on the floor a few inches from your body with your palms facing up. Keep your chin down. Stay in this position for two minutes.

It is essential that while lying in Savasana your attention is kept in the practice. Your mind should not wander about aimlessly but should be passively alert and aware. Keep your attention absorbed in the practice by observing a particular aspect, such as the effect that the postures have had on particular areas of your body. Do not extend your breath but observe, noting its quality and length. If parts of your body are tense, keep your attention focused on them and consciously relax them.

10.26

(j) Pranayama

1 Remain in Savasana.

2 Inhale slowly, filling your lungs from the top downwards. Observe the movement of your upper chest, ribs and abdomen. Count your breath mentally.

3 Exhale slowly, starting from the bottom, observing the movement of your abdomen, ribs and chest. Your abdomen can be contracted towards the end of the breath. Count the breath mentally and try to make the exhalation longer than the inhalation.

4 Repeat for between six and eighteen breaths, counting each breath on the fingers of one hand, as explained on page 146.

(k) Savasana — corpse pose

Remain lying in Savasana. And remember that it is essential that while lying in Savasana your attention is kept in the practice; your mind should not wander about aimlessly but should be passively alert and aware (see page 181).

Resumé

10.27

Savasana
2—3 minutes

Ekapada Urdhva Prasrta Padasana
4 × 2 breaths

Urdhva Prasrta Padasana
6 breaths

Cakravakasana
6 breaths

Vajrasana
6 breaths

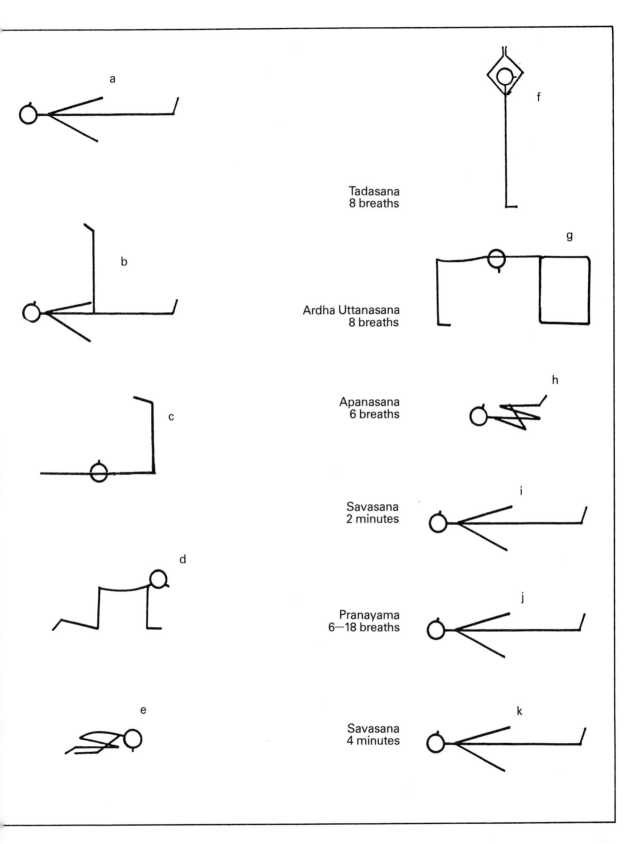

a

b

c

d

e

f

Tadasana
8 breaths

Ardha Uttanasana
8 breaths

g

Apanasana
6 breaths

h

Savasana
2 minutes

i

Pranayama
6–18 breaths

j

Savasana
4 minutes

k

Example 2 — A Vinyasa for Ardha Matsyendrasana

Explanatory notes

This is an example of a more demanding Vinyasa. The main posture is the twisting pose Ardha Matsyendrasana *(Fig. 10.28)* and, in order to help prepare for this asana, two other twisting postures are included in the sequence, Trikonasana and Jathara Parivrtti *(10.29g)*.

The Vinyasa *(Fig. 10.29)* begins with several breaths in Samasthiti (a), which is followed by a variation of Uttanasana (b) where your arms are swept behind your back to help prepare your shoulders for Ardha Matsyendrasana (i). This also warms up your body and prepares for Trikonasana (c) which itself prepares for the stronger twisting which takes place in Ardha Matsyendrasana.

Since your body has been twisted in Trikonasana, a forward-bending posture, Prasrta Pada Uttanasana (d), is needed to act as a counter-pose in order to help realign your organs and muscles. Utkatasana (e) acts as a counter-pose to Prasrta Pada Uttanasana, working your back in the opposite way, as well as releasing your legs which have been stretched in Uttanasana, Trikonasana and Prasrta Pada Uttanasana. Jathara Parivrtti (g), because it is a twisting posture, also helps prepare for Ardha Matsyendrasana, this being followed by Apanasana (h) which acts as a counter-pose.

The preparation for the main pose is now complete and the posture can be attempted (i). It is followed by Vajrasana (j) which acts as its counter-pose and is used dynamically, moving your arms, shoulders and legs.

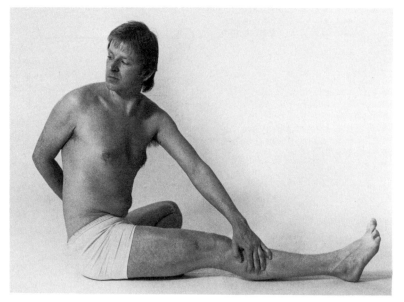

10.28

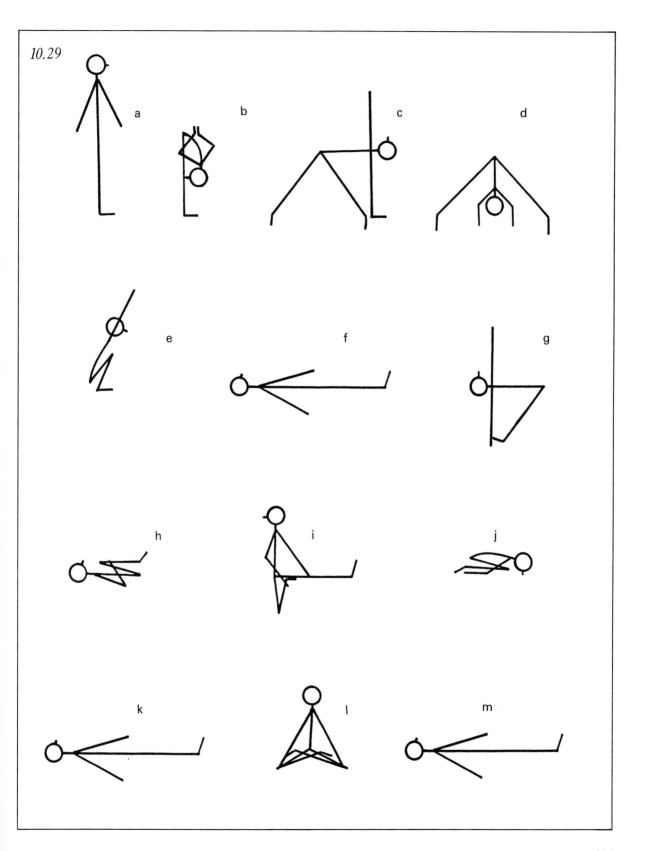

185

(a) Samasthiti — standing pose

10.30

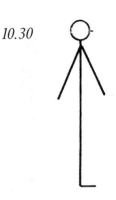

1 Stand upright, with your feet together a few inches apart but parallel. Your head should be bent down slightly.

2 Begin by turning your attention gradually towards the practice. Observe your breath and, as your attention becomes more centred, begin slowly to extend the breath, filling the upper part of your lungs first and working down. Make sure that your breath is even, calm, controlled and relaxed.

Stay for five to ten breaths until your mind is calm and in tune with the breath.

(b) Uttanasana — forward stretched pose

10.31

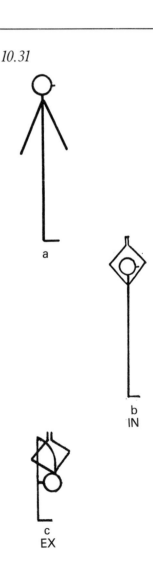

1 Stand in Samasthiti (a).

a

2 Inhaling, raise your arms above your head (b).

b
IN

3 Exhaling, bend forward, sweeping your arms behind your back (c).

c
EX

4 Inhaling, come up, sweeping your arms above your head as your body comes up (d).

Repeat for six breaths.

Avoid hunching your shoulders while going down into the posture.
If your legs and back are stiff, bend your knees while going down into the posture.
Observe the accumulative effect of working dynamically in the posture, and note if the inhalation or exhalation is harder to control.

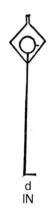

d
IN

(c) Trikonasana — triangle pose

10.32

1 Stand in Samasthiti (a).

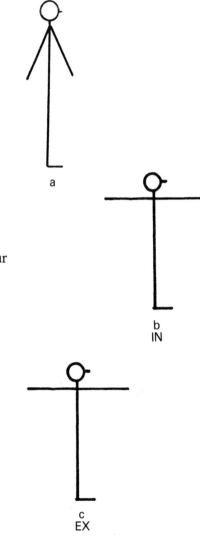

2 Inhaling, raise your arms to shoulder height (b). Keep your shoulder blades apart and your shoulders relaxed.

3 Exhale (c).

4 Inhaling, spread your legs 3—4 feet apart, with your feet parallel (d).

5 Exhaling, bend forward until your body is parallel to the floor (e).

6 Inhale (f).

7 Exhaling, twist sideways, taking your right hand towards your left foot (g). Keep your arms in line with each other and keep your right hip back.

8 Inhale (h).

9 Exhaling, turn your head upwards and look at your left hand (i).

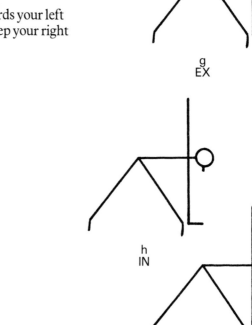

10 Stay in this position for six to eight breaths, turning your head upwards on the inhalation and turning it back towards the floor on the exhalation.

11 Repeat on the other side.

10.33

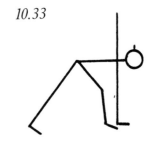

The twisting movement into the posture should come from the lower back. Avoid simply sweeping your lower arm across.

If, because of tightness in your legs, the twisting movement is very restricted, bend your knee *(Fig. 10.33)*.

To prevent your hips moving while twisting into the posture, occasionally work in the posture with your buttocks leaning against a wall.

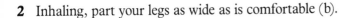

(d) *Prasrta Pada Uttanasana — stretch-leg forward-bend pose*

10.34

1 Stand in Samasthiti (a).

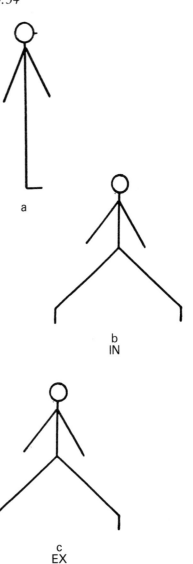

a

2 Inhaling, part your legs as wide as is comfortable (b).

b
IN

3 Exhale (c).

c
EX

4 Inhaling, raise your arms above your head (d).

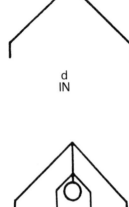

d
IN

5 Exhaling, bend forward placing your hands on the floor (e).

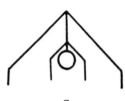

e
EX

6 Inhaling, look up, keeping your head and upper body raised so that only your fingertips remain on the floor (f).

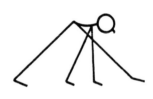

f
IN

7 Exhaling, lower your head and body towards the floor (g).

Repeat for six to eight breaths.

g
EX

10.35

If the posture is difficult it can be modified by placing your hands on a low stool *(Fig. 10.35)*.

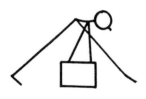

(e) Utkatasana — squatting pose

10.36

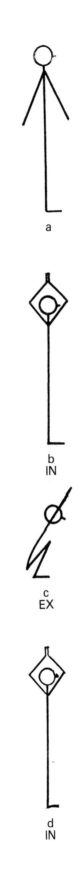

1 Stand upright in Samasthiti (a) with your feet together or a few inches apart.

2 Inhaling, raise your arms above your head and place the palms of your hands together (b).

3 Exhaling, bend your knees, lowering your body slowly until your buttocks nearly touch your calves, lowering your arms as you come down (c). Keep your heels on the floor.

4 Inhaling, come up, raising your arms above your head (d).

Repeat for four to six breaths.

If, because your heels are kept on the floor, you lose your balance, put a book or wooden block under your heels. Have your feet 6–8 inches apart. You will find the posture is more effective for working your ankle joints if your heels are supported in this way.

Try to keep your legs parallel as you move in the posture and observe if your legs have a tendency to come in or spread out as you move in the posture.

When coming up from the posture do not let all the movement come from your hips but work as much as possible on your upper back.

(f) Savasana — corpse pose

Lie down on your back, making sure your body is straight. Place your hands on the floor a few inches from your body, with the palms facing upwards. Keep your chin down.

It is essential that while lying in Savasana, you keep your attention in your practice (see page 183).

(g) Jathara Parivrtti — stomach twist

10.37

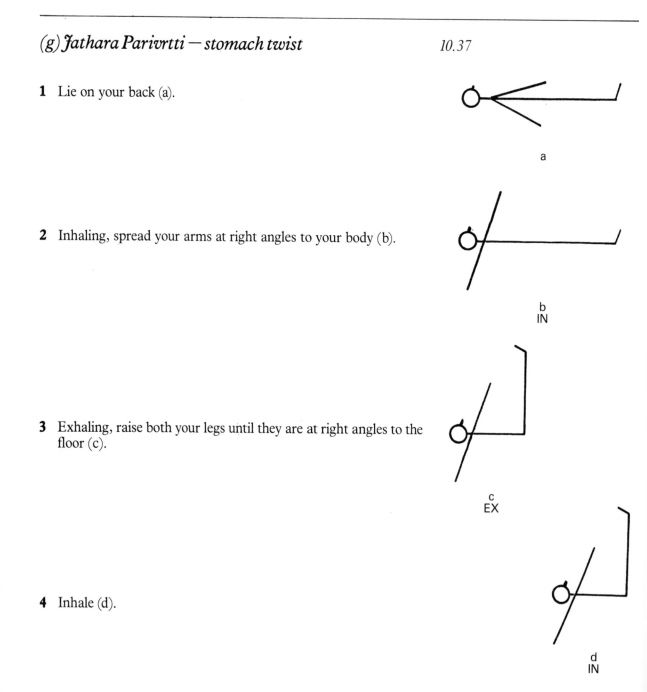

1 Lie on your back (a).

a

2 Inhaling, spread your arms at right angles to your body (b).

b
IN

3 Exhaling, raise both your legs until they are at right angles to the floor (c).

c
EX

4 Inhale (d).

d
IN

5 Exhaling, lower both your legs down towards your right hand. Try to keep your left shoulder on the floor (e).

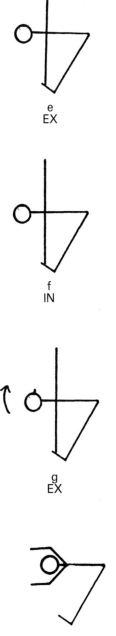

e
EX

6 Inhale (f).

f
IN

7 Exhaling, turn your head towards your left hand (g).

Stay in this position for eight breaths, turning your head back on each inhalation.

g
EX

Repeat on the other side.

If the posture is too vigorous for you, you can modify it by bending your knees or placing your feet on the floor away from your hands.

To intensify the effect of the posture you can inhale and sweep your arms along the floor, until the palms touch *(Fig. 10.38)*.

Observe how your breath is affected in this pose, noting its length and which part of your chest expands the most.

10.38

(h) Apanasana (counter-pose) — abdomen pose 10.39

1 Lying on your back, inhale (a).

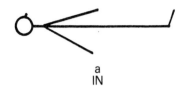

a
IN

2 Exhaling, bend your knees onto your abdomen and place your hands around your knees (b).

b
EX

3 Inhale (c).

c
IN

4 Exhaling, raise your head and move your forehead towards your knees (d).

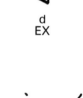

d
EX

5 Inhaling, lower your head to the floor, keeping your chin down (e).

Repeat for six breaths.

e
IN

Do not try to force your head and knees to touch; simply bring your head up as far as is comfortable.

(i) Ardha Matsyendrasana — half spine twist

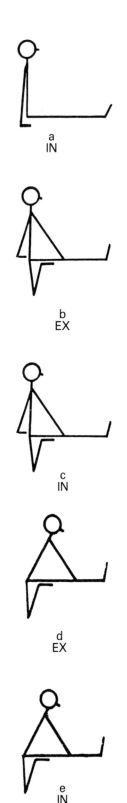

1 Sit on the floor with your legs straight and your back straight; inhale (a).

a
IN

2 Exhaling, bend your right leg and place your right foot on the inside of your left thigh (b). Keep your back straight and distribute your weight evenly on both of your buttocks.

b
EX

3 Inhaling, slightly arch your back (c).

c
IN

4 Exhaling, bend slightly forward and place the palm of your right hand on the outside of your left knee (d).

d
EX

5 Inhaling, straighten your back, slightly arching your lower back (e).

e
IN

6 Exhaling, turn your trunk and neck to the left and place your left arm behind your back and take hold of your right thigh (f).

Remain in this position for six to eight breaths.

Repeat on the other side.

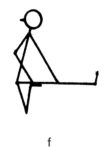

f

(j) Vajrasana — spine pose   10.41

1 Sit on your heels (a).

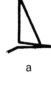

a

2 Inhaling, raise your arms above your head (b).

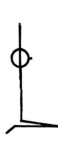

b
IN

3 Exhaling, bend forward, sweeping your arms behind your back with your hands resting on the floor by your heels (c).

c
EX

4 Inhaling, come up from the pose, sweeping your arms above your head (d).

Repeat for four breaths.

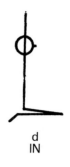

d
IN

If this posture is not comfortable for you, you can use Apanasana instead.
If your buttocks have a tendency to come up, put a cushion under your knees.

(k) Savasana — corpse pose

Lie down on your back. Inhale and carefully straighten your legs. Place your hands on the floor a few inches from your body, with the palms facing upwards. Keep your chin down. Rest for 5 minutes.
It is essential that while lying in Savasana you keep your attention in your practice. Your mind should not wander about aimlessly but should be passively alert and aware. Keep your attention absorbed in your practice by observing a particular aspect, such as the effect that the postures have had on particular areas of your body, or observe your breath, noting its quality and length. If parts of your body are tense, keep the attention focused on them and consciously relax them.

(l) Pranayama, Viloma Ujjayi — against the grain victorious

1 Choose a comfortable sitting posture, with the spine straight and chin slightly down (see pages 141–3).
2 Bend your first and second fingers so that they touch your palm.
3 Inhale slowly through your right nostril by blocking your left nostril with the thumb just below the point where the bone finishes and apply gentle pressure on your right nostril with the third finger so that there is a slight resistance. This gives you more control of your breath.
4 Exhale through both nostrils, controlling your breath at the throat (see page 151).
5 Inhale through your left nostril.
6 Keep the length of your inhalation and exhalation the same, e.g. 1:0:1:0:
   IN(6) : H(0) : EX (6) : H(0)
   or:
   IN(10) : H(0) : EX(10) : H(0)
7 Every six breaths increase the length of your breath by 2 or 4 seconds until you reach the comfortable limit of your capacity (see Table 10.1 for examples).
8 Finish the session by taking six shorter breaths with free inhalation and exhalation in Ujjayi.
9 Rest in either a sitting position or in Savasana.

Table 10.1 Examples of increasing lengths of breath in Viloma Ujjayi

IN	H	EX	H	Nos of breaths
6	0	6	0	6
8	0	8	0	6
10	0	10	0	6
Free breathing				6

or:

IN	H	EX	H	Nos of breaths
8	0	8	0	6
10	0	10	0	6
12	0	12	0	6
Free breathing				6

or:

IN	H	EX	H	Nos of breaths
6	0	6	0	6
12	0	12	0	6
18	0	18	0	12
Free breathing				6

or:

IN	H	EX	H	Nos of breaths
8	0	8	0	6
16	0	16	0	6
20	0	20	0	12
Free breathing				6

Resumé

10.42

Samasthit
6–8 breaths

Uttanasana
6 breaths

Trikonasana
6–8 breaths each side

Prasrta Pada Uttanasana
6–8 breaths

Utkatasana
6 breaths

Savasana
2 minutes

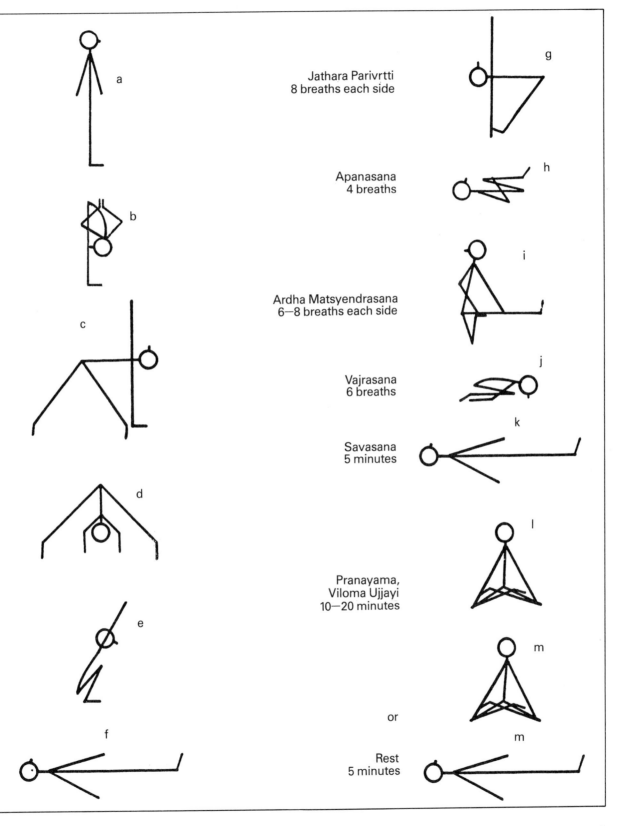

a

b

c

d

e

f

Jathara Parivrtti
8 breaths each side

g

Apanasana
4 breaths

h

Ardha Matsyendrasana
6–8 breaths each side

i

Vajrasana
6 breaths

j

Savasana
5 minutes

k

Pranayama,
Viloma Ujjayi
10–20 minutes

l

m

or

m

Rest
5 minutes

Example 3 — A Vinyasa for Sarvangasana

Explanatory notes

This Vinyasa, with Sarvangasana *(Fig. 10.43)* as its main pose, is again fairly demanding. The first posture in the Vinyasa *(Fig. 10.44)*, Samasthiti (a), is used with several slow breaths and helps to prepare mentally and physically for the Vinyasa, while Tadasana (b) warms your body, helps expand your chest and deepens the breath.

Uttanasana (c) is used both dynamically and statically. Used dynamically, it helps to warm up your body; used statically, it stretches the back of your legs and accustoms your head to a downward position. Adhomukha Svanasana (d) prepares your shoulders, arms and wrists and is also useful because, as in Sarvangasana, your head is inverted.

Vajrasana (e) used dynamically acts as a counter-pose for the three previous postures, releasing your shoulders, arms and legs. A short rest in Savasana (f) may then be necessary for some students, depending on how many breaths the previous postures have been held for.

Dvipada Pitham (g) helps prepare your neck for Sarvangasana (i) which can be held for between twelve and twenty-four breaths. Beginners should start with six breaths, gradually increasing the number over a period of several weeks. Sarvangasana is followed by a few breaths in Savasana (j).

Bhujangasana (k) acts as one of the best counter-postures to Sarvangasana for a number of reasons. Firstly it acts as a counter-balance to the neck by allowing free movement in the oppposite direction. It is a better counter-pose than Matsyasana *(Fig. 10.45)*, where the position of the neck is rigid. In Bhujangasana the neck, arms and shoulders can move, which is helpful as these areas are static in Sarvangasana. Your back, which has a tendency to become concave in Sarvangasana, is stretched in the opposite direction. Vajrasana (l) acts as a counter-pose to Bhujangasana, and the Vinyasa finishes with a rest in Savasana.

The breath in the principal postures can be with a longer exhalation, as preparation for a longer exhalation in Anuloma Ujjayi Pranayama. In this Pranayama the breath is inhaled through the nostrils and controlled with the fingers on the exhalation. This makes it easier to work with a longer exhalation, which will generally have a relaxing effect.

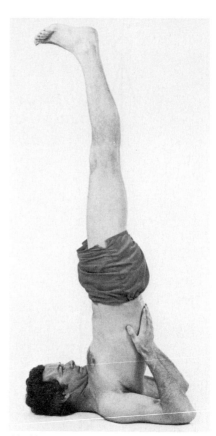

10.43

10.45

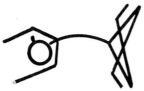

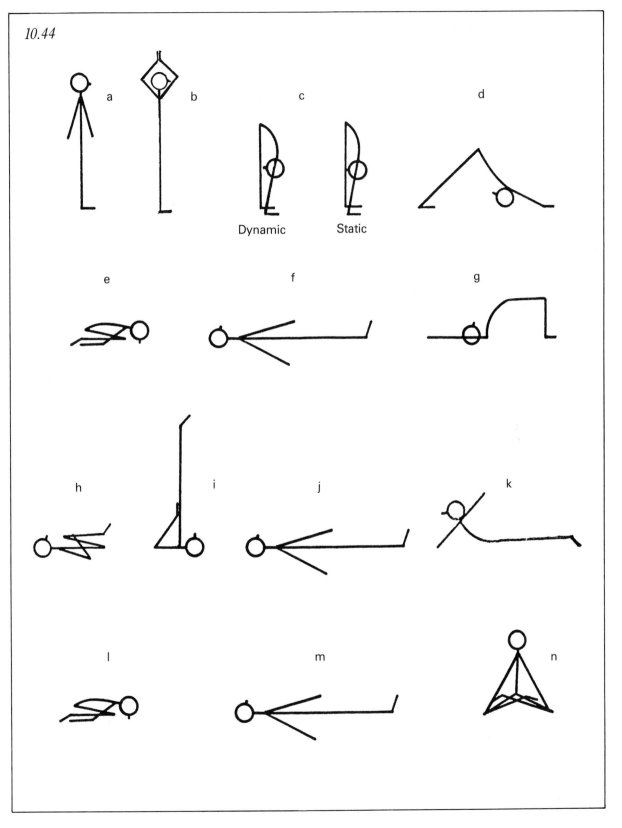

a

b

c

d

Dynamic   Static

e

f

g

h

i

j

k

l

m

n

(a) Samasthiti — standing pose

1 Stand upright with your feet together or a few inches apart, but parallel. Your head should be tilted slightly downwards.
2 Begin by turning your attention gradually towards the practice. Observe your breath and, as your attention becomes more centred, begin slowly to extend the breath, filling the upper part of your lungs first and working down. Make sure that the breath is even, calm, controlled and relaxed.
3 Stay in this position for five to ten breaths until your mind is calm and in tune with the breath.

10.46

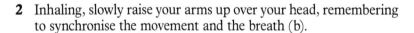

(b) Tadasana — palm tree pose

10.47

1 Stand upright with your feet together or a few inches apart (a).

a

2 Inhaling, slowly raise your arms up over your head, remembering to synchronise the movement and the breath (b).

b
IN

3 Exhaling, lower your arms to your sides (c), again synchronising the movement and the breath (see Chapter 5).

c
EX

Repeat for six to eight breaths.

Your arms can be raised and lowered either sideways or frontwards or in combinations of both. By doing this your shoulder joint is rotated in different ways.

Keep your chin down.

When your arms are raised, pull your arms back and work your upper back.

Avoid hollowing your lower back as your arms are raised.

If your arm movement is restricted or there is stiffness or tension in your neck and/or shoulders, bend your elbows.

(c) Uttanasana — forward stretched pose

10.48

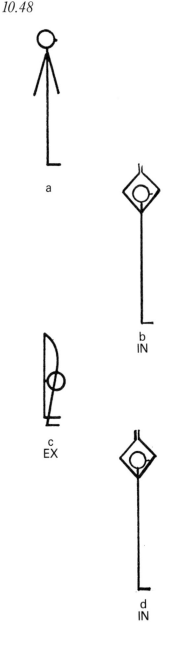

a

b
IN

c
EX

d
IN

1 Stand in Samasthiti (a).

2 Inhaling, raise your arms above your head (b).

3 Exhaling, bend forward (c). While moving into the posture, keep your arms back, your chest open and slightly hollow your lower back.

4 Inhaling, come up slowly, lifting your arms first, and working along your spine (d).

Repeat for six breaths.

6 On the sixth exhalation stay down in the posture (e).

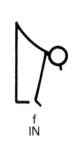

e
EX

7 Inhaling, lift up your head, shoulders and upper back so only your fingertips are touching the floor (f).

Repeat for six breaths.

f
IN

Compare the effect of working dynamically and statically on:

1 your legs;
2 your lower back;
3 your breath.

(d) Adhomukha Svanasana – downward-facing dog pose   10.49

1 Stand in Samasthiti (a).

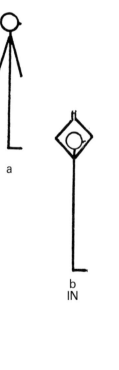

a

2 Inhaling, raise your arms above your head (b).

b
IN

3 Exhaling, bend forward into Uttanasana (see page 203) and place your hands on the floor (c). Bend your knees if your hands do not reach the floor easily.

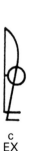

c
EX

4 Inhale and step back, one leg at a time (d). The distance will vary according to how tall you are and how you want to use the pose, but it should be roughly 3–3½ feet.

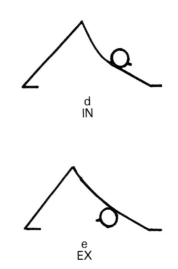

d
IN

5 Exhaling, move your head towards the floor (e).

e
EX

Repeat for eight breaths.

There are a great many modifications to this posture *(Fig. 10.50)*. One which is particularly useful is to lift your heels and bend your knees (a). This allows more movement in your spine, which should *not* be rounded (b). The distance between your hands and feet can be varied (c, d) according to which part of your body needs to be worked.

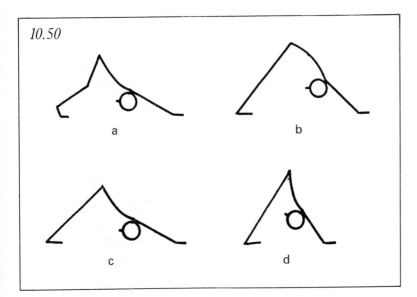

10.50

a

b

c

d

(e) Vajrasana (counter-pose) — spine pose

10.51

1 Inhaling, come down from Adhomukha Svanasana by placing your knees on the floor (a).
2 Exhaling, place your buttocks on your heels, bringing your arms to your sides and placing your forehead on the floor (b).

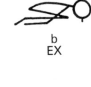

a
IN

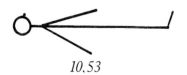

b
EX

Stay in this posture with relaxed breathing for six to eight breaths.

While resting in the counter-pose, keep your attention on the asana and observe the effects of the previous posture.

If this posture is not comfortable for you, use Apanasana (Fig. 10.52) instead.

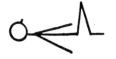

10.52

(f) Savasana — corpse pose

Lie on your back. Place your hands on the floor a few inches from your body with your palms facing upwards (Fig. 10.53). Keep your chin down. Rest for 5 minutes.

It is essential that while lying in Savasana you keep your attention in your practice (see page 181).

10.53

(g) Dvipada Pitham — desk pose

10.54

1 Lie on your back and inhale (a).

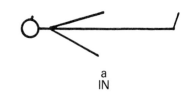

a
IN

2 Exhaling slowly, bend your legs, placing your feet on the floor close to your buttocks (b). Have your feet parallel and about 6—8 inches apart.

b
EX

3 Inhaling, lift your buttocks off the floor and take your arms over your head, synchronising both movements (c).

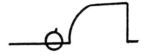

c
IN

4 Exhaling, lower your buttocks onto the floor and bring your arms to your side (d). Synchronise these two movements.

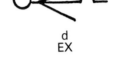

d
EX

5 Repeat for four breaths, dynamically.

6 Inhaling, go up into the posture and stay for four breaths. Keep your arms by your side (e) and lift your buttocks a little higher on each inhalation.

e
Static

Try working in this posture with your feet and knees together and note the effect this has.

(h) Apanasana (counter-pose) — abdomen pose

10.55

1 Lie on your back with your chin down slightly and your arms by your sides (a). Inhale.

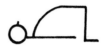

a
IN

2 Exhaling slowly, bend your knees and place both legs on your abdomen with your hands around your knees (b). Do not try to force your knees onto your chest. Keep your lower back on the floor.

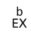

b
EX

3 Stay in this position for six breaths.

4 Inhaling, straighten your legs and place your arms by your sides (c).

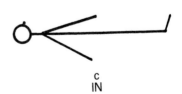

c
IN

207

(i) Sarvangasana — shoulder stand

10.56

1 Lie on your back with your chin down, and your arms by your sides, palms down (a). Inhale.

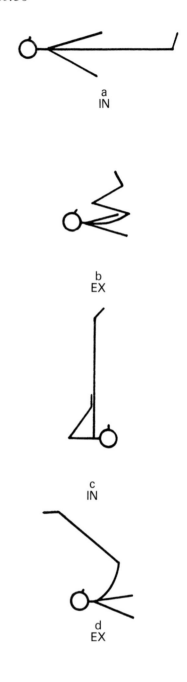

2 Exhaling, *slowly* raise your legs and lift your buttocks from the floor (b).

3 Inhaling, straighten your body and support your back by placing your hands on your lower back (c).

4 Stay in this position for between eight and sixteen breaths.

5 Exhaling, slowly come down from the posture by bending and lowering your legs over your head (d).

6 Inhaling place your arms on the floor and bring your legs and body down to the floor (e). The movement should be slow and controlled, and your head should be kept on the floor.

Do not attempt this posture without proper supervision.

Observe the quality and length of the breath. See how your breath changes with your upper chest restricted.

Observe which parts of your body become tired as the posture is held and see if alteration of the Vinyasa can help maintain the posture for a longer period.

(j) Savasana (counter-pose) — corpse pose

Inhale and carefully straighten your legs onto the floor. Place your hands on the floor a few inches from your body with your palms facing up *(Fig. 10.57)*. Keep your chin down.

It is essential that while lying in Savasana you keep your attention in your practice (see page 181).

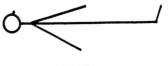

10.57

(k) Bhujangasana — cobra pose

10.58

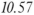

1 Lie face down, with your arms at your side (a).

a

2 Inhaling, raise your head and shoulders and sweep your arms sideways until they are at right-angles to your body (b).

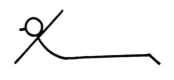

b
IN

3 Exhale slowly and lower your head, shoulders and arms onto the floor, sweeping your arms back to your sides (c).

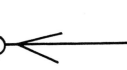

c
EX

Repeat for four to eight breaths.

Do not hunch your shoulders as you move into the posture, but keep your shoulder blades apart.

If your shoulders are tense, bend your elbows.

209

(l) Apanasana (counter-pose) — abdomen pose

10.59

1 Turn over on to your back and inhale (a).

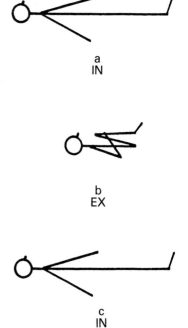

a
IN

2 Exhaling, slowly bend your knees and place both legs on your abdomen with your hands around your knees (b). Do not try to force your knees onto your chest. Keep your lower back on the floor.

Stay in this position for six breaths.

b
EX

3 Inhale and straighten your legs (c).

c
IN

Apanasana is the counter-posture to Bhujangasana. While holding the posture, keep your attention in the practice, observing the effects that the previous postures have had.

(m) Savanasana — corpse pose

Place your hands on the floor a few inches from your body with your palms facing up *(Fig. 10.60)*. Keep your chin down. Rest for 5 minutes.

It is essential that while lying in Savasana you keep your attention in your practice (see page 181).

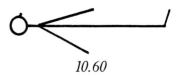

10.60

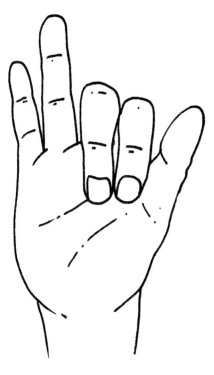

(n) Pranayama, Anuloma Ujjayi — with the grain victorious

1. Choose a comfortable sitting posture, with your spine straight and your chin down slightly (see pages 141–3).
2. Bend your first and second fingers down so that they touch your palm.
3. Inhale, slowly, through both nostrils, controlling your breath at the throat.
4. Exhale, slowly, through your left nostril by blocking your right nostril with your thumb just below the point where the bone finishes. As you exhale through your left nostril apply a gentle pressure with your third finger so that there is a slight resistance. This gives the quality of the breath much more refinement.
5. Inhale slowly through both nostrils, controlling the breath at your throat.
6. Exhale slowly through your right nostril.
7. Use one of the ratios in Table 10.2.
8. Either remain sitting or lie down in Savasana for 5–10 minutes.

Table 10.2 Examples of Rechaka ratios in Anuloma Ujjayi, where the emphasis is on longer exhalation

	IN	H	EX	H	Nos of breaths
	6	0	12	0	6
	8	0	16	0	12
	6	0	12	0	6
or:					
	8	0	16	0	6
	10	0	20	0	12
	8	0	16	0	6

Keep your attention focused within the practice. Observe very carefully the quality of the breath from the beginning to the end of each breath. Avoid trying to extend the breath too much and remember that its quality is of far more importance than its length.

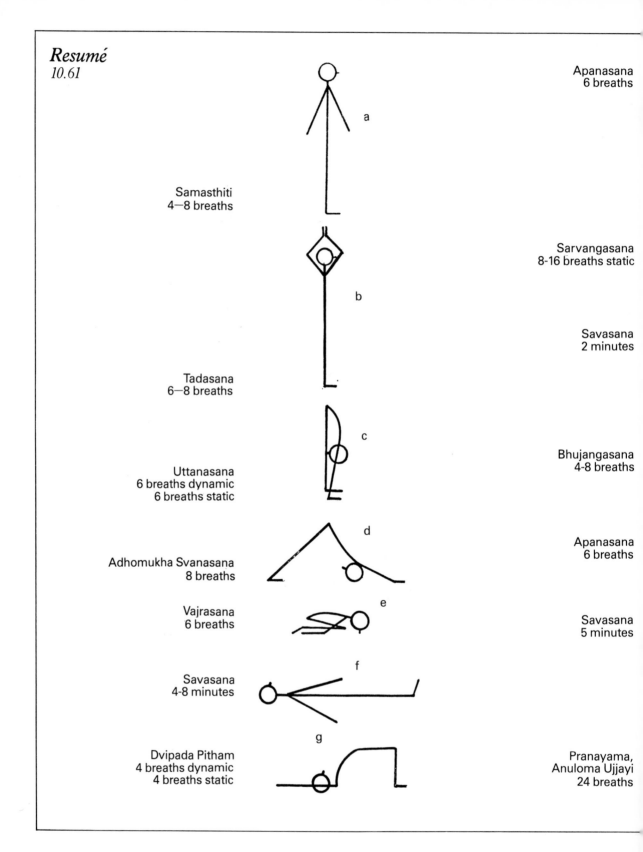

Resumé
10.61

Samasthiti
4—8 breaths

Tadasana
6—8 breaths

Uttanasana
6 breaths dynamic
6 breaths static

Adhomukha Svanasana
8 breaths

Vajrasana
6 breaths

Savasana
4-8 minutes

Dvipada Pitham
4 breaths dynamic
4 breaths static

Apanasana
6 breaths

Sarvangasana
8-16 breaths static

Savasana
2 minutes

Bhujangasana
4-8 breaths

Apanasana
6 breaths

Savasana
5 minutes

Pranayama,
Anuloma Ujjayi
24 breaths

a
b
c
d
e
f
g

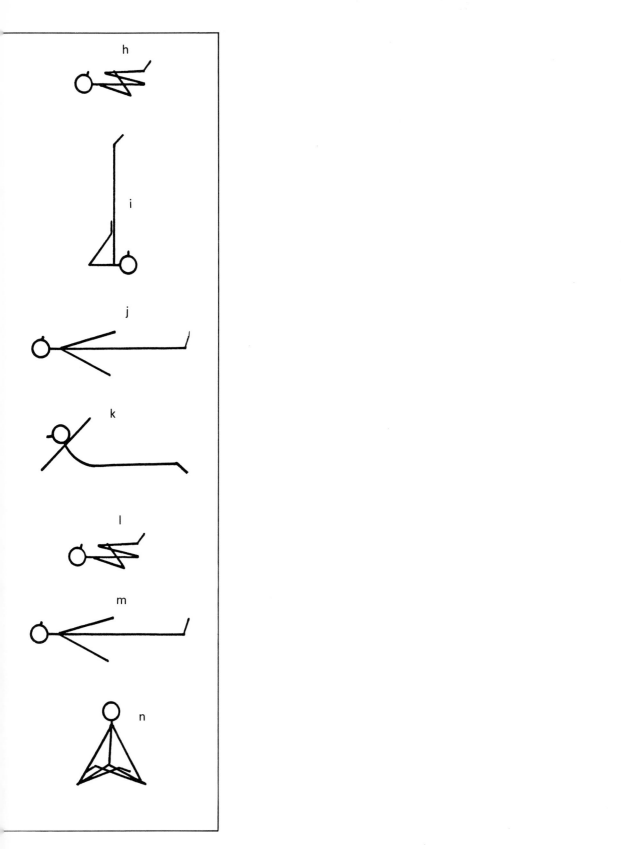

h

i

j

k

l

m

n

213

Example 4 — A Vinyasa for Ustrasana

Explanatory notes

This is the most strenuous of the four examples. The main asana is Ustrasana *(Fig. 10.62)* which has been modified so the hands are placed on a wall. This makes the posture considerably stronger, and so thorough preparation will be needed. The posture should not be attempted without supervision.

The Vinyasa *(Fig. 10.63)* begins with a few breaths in Samasthiti (a) and is followed by Parsva Uttanasana (b) used dynamically, which warms up the body and, because it is an asymmetrical posture, helps prepare for Virabhadrasana (c), which is also asymmetrical. Virabhadrasana is used because it is a back-bending posture which helps prepare for Ustrasana (j). Since Virabhadrasana is a back bend, its counter-pose needs to be a forward bend; in this sequence Uttanasana (d) is used statically, followed by Utkatasana (e), which is included to act as a counter-pose for the legs. The standing sequence is followed by a short rest in Savasana (f).

Salabhasana (g) is a moderate back-bend and helps prepare for a stronger back-bend, Dhanurasana (h). Dhanurasana in its turn helps prepare the shoulders and lower back for the main pose. Salabhasana and Dhanurasana are followed by Vajrsana (i), which acts as a mild counter-pose.

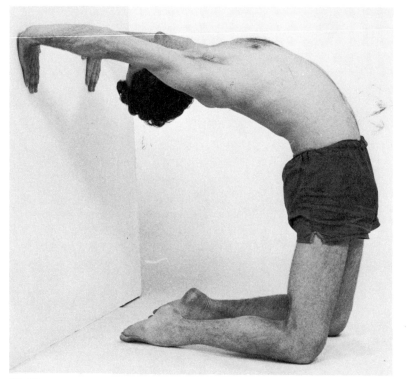

10.62

214

The preparation for Ustrasana (j) is now complete, and it should be possible to hold the pose for a number of breaths without any strain. Vajrasana (k) is used again, dynamically, as a counter-pose after the main posture, this time with arm movements to remove any strain in the shoulders and arms. The sequence ends with a rest in Savasana (l).

During Parsva Uttanasana, Virabhadrasana, Uttanasana, Salabhasana, Dhanurasana and Ustrasana, attempt to work with a 1:0:1:0 ratio in order to help prepare for the Pranayama (m) in Nadisodhana, where the lengths of the inhalation and exhalation are extended.

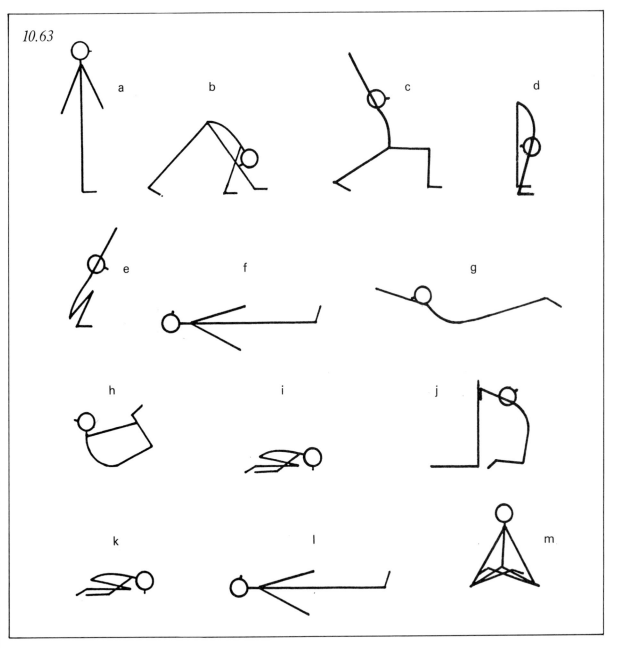

10.63

a   b   c   d

e   f   g

h   i   j

k   l   m

(a) Samasthiti — standing pose

See page 202.

(b) Parsva Uttanasana — side forward bend

10.64

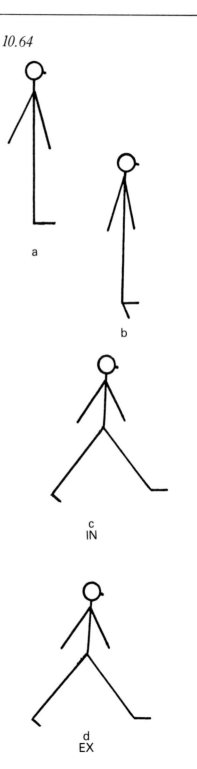

1 Stand in Samasthiti (a).

2 Turn your right foot to 45° (b).

3 Inhaling, step forward 3 feet with your left leg. The distance between your feet will vary according to your height and the intended effect of the posture. Bring your right hip round and keep the weight on your right heel (c).

4 Exhale (d).

5 Inhaling, raise your arms above your head (e). Bend your elbows if there is any tension in your back, shoulders or lower back.

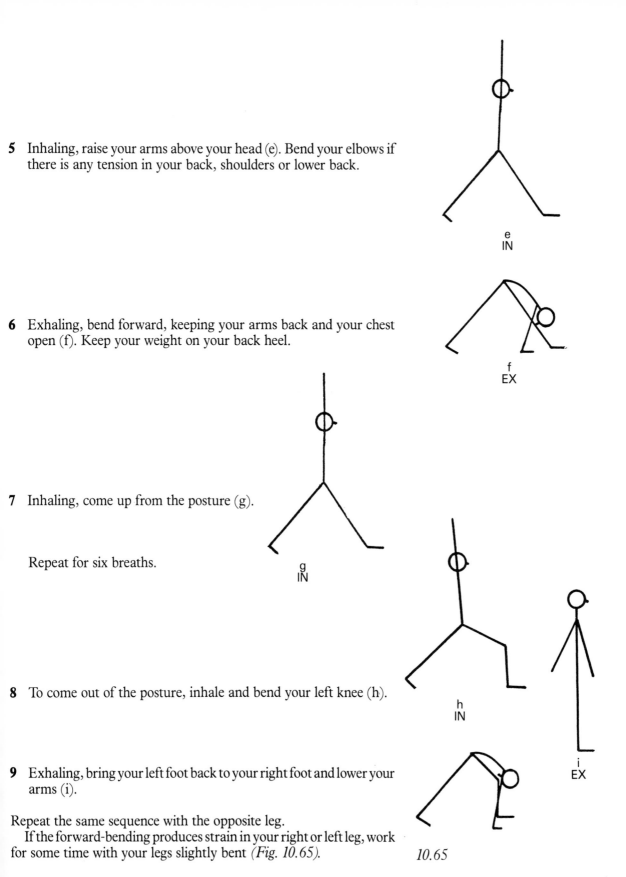

e
IN

6 Exhaling, bend forward, keeping your arms back and your chest open (f). Keep your weight on your back heel.

f
EX

7 Inhaling, come up from the posture (g).

Repeat for six breaths.

g
IN

8 To come out of the posture, inhale and bend your left knee (h).

h
IN

i
EX

9 Exhaling, bring your left foot back to your right foot and lower your arms (i).

Repeat the same sequence with the opposite leg.
    If the forward-bending produces strain in your right or left leg, work for some time with your legs slightly bent *(Fig. 10.65)*.

10.65

(c) Virabhadrasana — warrior pose

10.66

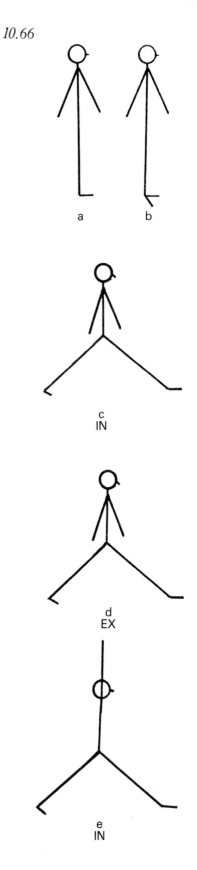

1 Stand in Samasthiti (a).

2 Turn your right foot to 45° (b).

3 Inhaling, step forward 4–4½ feet with your left leg (c). The distance between your feet will vary according to your height.

4 Exhale (d).

5 Inhaling, raise your arms above your head (e).

6 Exhaling, bend your left knee so your thigh is parallel to the floor and your lower leg from your foot to your knee is at right-angles to the floor (f).

7 Inhaling, open your chest, lean back slightly, arching your back (g).

8 Stay in this position for four to six slow breaths.

9 Exhaling, bring your left foot back to your right foot (h).

10 Inhale (i).

11 Exhaling, lower your arms (j).

Repeat on the other side.

    Because this is a demanding posture the length and quality of your breath may change. Carefully observe your breath and see if either the inhalation or exhalation is harder to control.

    Compare working on the left and right sides of your body.

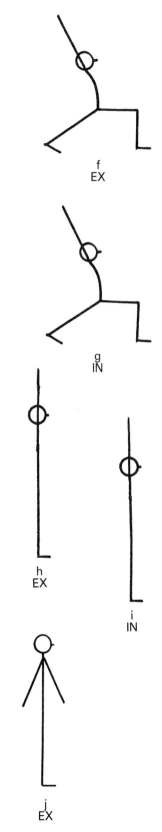

f
EX

g
IN

h
EX

i
IN

j
EX

219

(d) Uttanasana — forward stretched pose

10.67

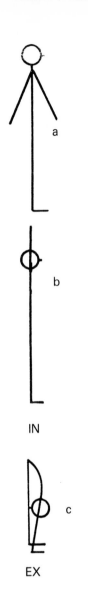

1 Stand in Samasthiti (a).

2 Inhaling, raise your arms above your head (b).

3 Exhale, bend forward, keep your arms back, your chest open and your lower back slightly hollow. Place your hands on the floor (c).

Stay in the posture for six breaths.

This posture can be modified by bending your knees. Although the full effect of stretching your legs is lost, there is considerably more movement in your lower back, and if you have a stiff lower back, this modification is very useful.

Avoid hunching your back and shoulders as you move into the posture.

(e) Utkatasana — squatting pose

10.68

1 Stand upright in Samasthiti, with your feet together or a few inches apart (a).

2 Inhaling, raise your arms above your head, placing the palms of your hands together (b).

b

IN

3 Exhaling, bend your knees, lowering your body slowly until your buttocks nearly touch your calves. Keep your arms above your head as you come down (c). Keep your heels on the floor.

c

EX

d

4 Inhaling, come up, keeping your arms above your head (d).

IN

Repeat this movement for four to six breaths.

If, because your heels are kept on the floor you lose your balance, put a book or wedge under your heels and have your feet 6—8 inches apart. The posture is more effective for working your ankle joint if your heel is supported.

When coming up from the posture do not let all the movement come from your hips but work as much as possible on your upper back.

(f) Savasana — corpse pose

Lie down on your back and carefully straighten your legs onto the floor. Place your hands on the floor a few inches from your body with your palms facing up. Keep your chin down and your eyes closed. Remain in this position for one to two minutes.

It is essential that while lying in Savasana you keep your attention in your practice (see page 181).

(g) Salabhasana — locust pose

10.69

1 Lie face down with your arms above your head and with your palms together. To ensure that your legs are kept together put a thin book between your knees (a) and observe the effect that keeping your knees together has on your back.

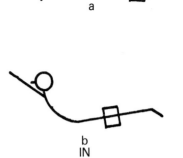

a

2 Inhaling, lift your arms, head and upper body and your legs. Keep your thighs and knees together (b).

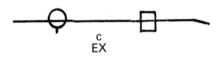

b
IN

3 Exhaling, lower your arms and upper body and legs back onto the floor (c).

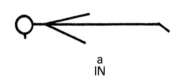

c
EX

Repeat this movement for four to eight breaths.
    Do not hunch your shoulders. If they are tense, bend your elbows.

(h) Dhanurasana — bow pose

10.70

1 Lie on your stomach. Inhale (a).

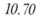

a
IN

2 Exhaling, bend both your legs and take hold of your ankles with your hands (b).

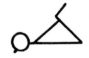

b
EX

3 Inhaling, lift your head and shoulders and pull your feet away from your body (c).

c
IN

4 Exhaling, lower your head and shoulders back onto the floor (d).

Repeat this movement for six breaths.
　The effect of this posture can be varied by keeping the thighs on the floor.

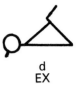

d
EX

(i) Vajrasana (counter-pose) — spine pose　　　　10.71

1 Sit on your heels (a).

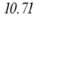

a

2 Inhaling, raise your arms above your head (b).

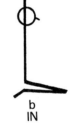

b
IN

3 Exhaling, bend forward, sweeping your arms behind your back with your hands resting on the floor by your heels (c).

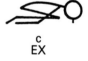

c
EX

Stay in this position for four to six breaths.

(j) Ustrasana (modified) — camel pose

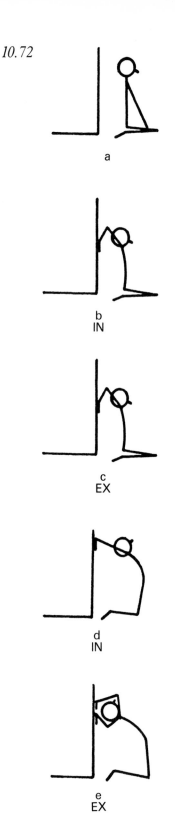

1 Sit on your heels with your knees 12—16 inches apart and your heels 6—8 inches from a wall (a).

2 Inhaling, raise your arms above your head and place your palms against the wall, with your fingers pointing towards the floor (b).

3 Exhale.

4 Inhaling, lift your buttocks off your heels and arch your back (d).

5 Exhaling, bend your elbows and lower your body a few inches (e).

6 Inhale and gradually straighten your arms again (f).

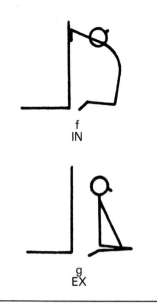

f
IN

7 Repeat this movement for four to eight breaths.

8 Exhaling, come down from the pose and sit on your heels (g).

g
EX

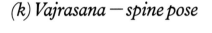

(k) Vajrasana — spine pose

10.73

1 Sit on your heels (a).

a

2 Inhaling, raise your arms above your head (b).

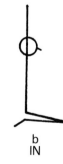

b
IN

3 Exhaling, bend forward sweeping your arms behind your back with your hands resting on the floor by your heels (c).

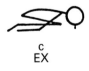

c
EX

Repeat this movement for six to eight breaths.
Observe the effect of Vajrasana on your lower back. If your lower back feels stiff remain statically in the pose for six to eight breaths.

225

(l) Savasana — corpse pose

Lie down on your back and carefully straighten your body. Place your hands on the floor a few inches from your body, with your palms facing up. Keep your chin down.

It is essential that while lying in Savasana you keep your attention in the practice (see page 183).

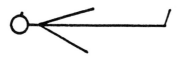

(m) Pranayama Nadisodhana — channel to clean

1 Choose a comfortable sitting position.
2 Follow the directions for controlling your breath with your fingers as described on page 151.
3 Inhale through your right nostril, controlling the flow of air by partially blocking the nostril with your finger or thumb, and completely blocking your left nostril.
4 Exhale through your left nostril, controlling the flow by partially blocking the nostril and completely blocking your right nostril.
5 Inhale through your left nostril, continuing to control the breath with your fingers.
6 Exhale through your right nostril.
7 Take six breaths using a 1:0:1:0 ratio.
8 After six breaths, retain the breath after the inhalation for 4 seconds. Every six breaths increase the length of retention by 4—6 seconds until you reach a comfortable maximum.
9 Complete the Pranayama by taking six breaths with free breathing, without retention and without counting the breath or trying to extend it.
10 Rest either in a sitting posture or in Savasana for 5 minutes.

Audio and video tapes of classes are available from the author.

Samasthiti
8 breaths

Parsva Uttanasana
6 × 2 breaths

Virabhadrasana
6 × 2 breaths

Uttanasana
6 breaths

Utkatasana
6 breaths

Savasana
2 minutes

Salabhasana
4-8 breaths

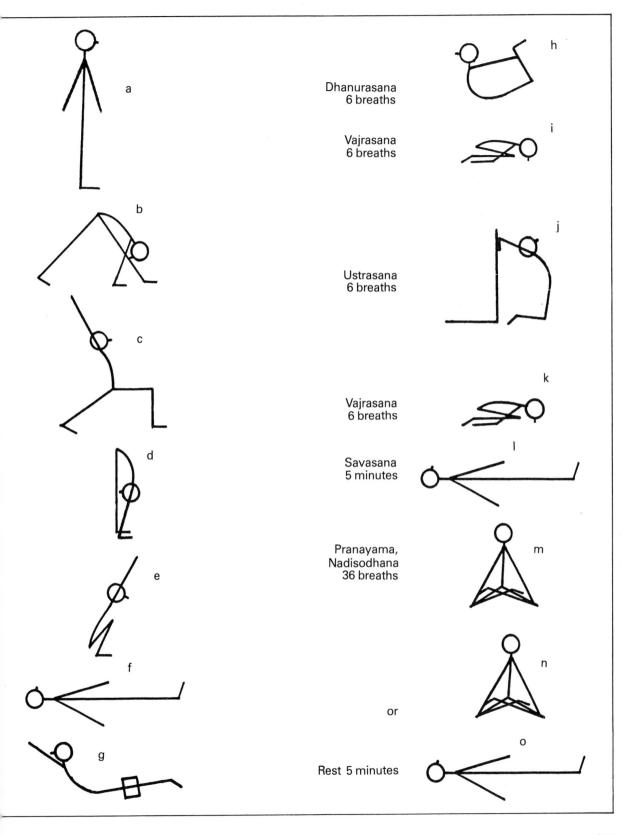

a

b

c

d

e

f

g

Dhanurasana
6 breaths

h

Vajrasana
6 breaths

i

Ustrasana
6 breaths

j

Vajrasana
6 breaths

k

Savasana
5 minutes

l

Pranayama,
Nadisodhana
36 breaths

m

n

or

o

Rest 5 minutes

227

Information about this approach to yoga is available from pupils of Desikachas at:

Viniyoga
134, BD Sauveniere
B 4000 Liege
Belgium

Viniyoga
c/o Marta Artigas
Barcelona 30
Granollers
Spain

Viniyoga
c/o Paul Harvey
48 Devonshire Buildings
Bath BA2 4SU
Great Britain

Viniyoga
c/o Chizuko Iwakiri Steinman
7 Miyanoshita, Daikakuji
Monsen, Saga, Ukyo-Ku
Kyoto
Japan 616

Viniyoga
2, Rue de Valois
75001 Paris
France

Viniyoga
c/o Malek Daouk
13, Av. Mon-Loisir
CH 1006 Lausanne
Switzerland

Viniyoga
c/o Peter Hersnack
Hesselo 33
2 T.V. DK 2100
Denmark

Viniyoga
America
1258 Mansfield Av.
N.E. Atlanta GA 30307
U.S.A.

GLOSSARY

Adhomukha   Face down.

Adhomuka Svanasana   Downward facing down dog pose. The posture resembles a dog stretching, with its back legs straight and head lowered (Fig. 1.4).

Antara   Within, interior.

Antah Kumbhaka   Suspension of the breath after the inhalation.

Anuloma   With the grain.

Apana   One of the five subdivisions of the pranic energy. It is primarily responsible for digestion and elimination.

Apanasana   Lower abdomen pose (Fig. 2.11).

Ardha   Half. Often used as a prefix to a classical posture when a variation is used holding the posture halfway, e.g. Ardha Uttanasana (Fig. 5.37).

Ardha Matsyendrasana   A sitting, twisting posture (Fig. 1.8) named after a yogi Matyandra.

Ardha Uttanasana   Name of a variation of Uttanasana, where the trunk is held halfway down to the floor (Fig. 10.24).

Ayama   To stretch, to control. The last part of the word Pranayama.

Bahya   External.

Bahya Kumbhaka   Suspending the breathing after the exhalation.

Bastrika   Bellows, furnace. A type of Pranayama where the breath is forced in and out very quickly.

Bedhana   To pierce, to penetrate.

Bhagirathasana   A posture named after King Bhagiratha, who did a penance of standing on one leg (Fig. 5.44).

Bhujangasana   *Bhujan* means a snake or serpent. The posture resembles a snake just before it attacks (Fig. 1.3 and 4.9).

Cakravakasana   Goose pose (Fig. 2.8).

Catuspadapitham   Four leg support. A posture where the feet and hands support the body (Fig. 2.30).

Chandra   Moon.

Danda   Rod or stick.

Dandasana   A posture where the back is held very straight like a rod (Fig. 7.2a).

Dhanurasana   Bow posture, named because it resembles the shape of a bow (Fig. 1.33).

Dvipada Pitham   Two feet support. A posture where the body is supported by the feet (Fig. 2.7).

Eka   One.

Ekapada   One foot. Used as a prefix to name variations of classical postures where one foot or leg is held in a different position from the classical position, e.g. *Ekapada Dvipadapitham* (Fig. 5.13b), *Ekapada Uttanasana* (Fig. 5.46), *Ekapada Urdhva Dhanurasana* (Fig. 1.28).

Halasana   Plough posture, named because it resembles a plough (Fig. 2.22).

Janu   Knee.

Janu Sirsasana   A posture where the head is lowered to the knee (Fig. 1.37).

Jathara Parivrtti *Jathara* = abdomen, *Parivrtti* = twist. A posture where the abdomen is twisted by rotating the legs to one side (Fig. 1.23f).

Kapotasana Pigeon pose, so called because the chest is expanded like a pigeon (Fig. 1.35).

Kona Angle.

Krauncasana Heron posture, named because the outstretched leg resembles the shape of a heron's head (Fig. 2.12).

Mahamudra *Mahe* = great, *Mudra* = seal (Fig. 5.42).

Maricyasana A twisting posture, named after a sage, Maricy, son of the creator, Brahma (Fig. 2.32).

Matsyasana Fish pose (Fig. 10.45).

Matsyendrasana A posture named after the yogi, Matsyendra (Fig. 1.8 shows Ardha Matsyendrasana).

Mukha Face, head.

Nadi A channel through which the prana flows in the body.

Nadisodhana A type of alternate-nostril breathing, where the breath is inhaled and exhaled through alternate nostrils.

Pada Foot, leg.

Padmasana Lotus posture, traditionally considered an important posture for Manayana and meditation (Fig. 1.31).

Parsva Side.

Parsva Uttanasana A posture where one side of the body is stretched, then the other side (Fig. 1.25).

Pascimatanasana A posture which stretches the back of the body (Fig. 1.6).

Patanjali Considered to be the author of the yoga sutras, the text of four chapters describing different aspects of yoga.

Prana Life force, energy, breath.

Prasrta Spread.

Prasrta Pada Uttanasana A forward-bending posture where the legs are spread wide apart (Fig. 2.16).

Pratiloma Neither with nor against the grain.

Purvatanasana *Purva* means east. Traditionally postures were practiced facing the rising sun, so the front of the body faces east. Purvottanasana stretches the front of the body (Fig. 7.16)

Salabhasana Locust posture (Fig. 1.14).

Samasthiti Standing at attention (Fig. 10.46).

Sama-vrtti Equal; inhalation and exhalation and retention in pranayama.

Sarvangasana *Sarva* = all, *Anga* = limbs, body. A posture which benefits the whole body (Fig. 1.10).

Savasana *Sava* means corpse. A posture for relaxation used during and after a series of postures (Fig. 2.39).

Siddhasana A sitting posture suitable for pranayama and meditation (Fig. 9.5).

Sirsasana Headstand (Fig. 1.12).

Sodhana To cleanse.

Sthira Stable, firm, one of the qualities that should be present in a posture.

Sukha   At ease.

Sukhasana   Comfortable sitting pose (Fig. 9.6).

Supta   Lying, sleep.

Supta Ekapada Padangusthasana   A lying posture where one foot is held (Fig. 7.8).

Surya   Sun.

Tadasana   Straight face, posture of the arms raised above the head (Fig. 5.7).

Tiryangmukha Ekapada Pascimatanasana   A posture where one leg is bent back and the head is placed on the knee (Fig. 6.26.)

Trikonasana   Three-angle pose. A standing posture with two principal variations, one a side stretch and one a twisting variation (Fig. 1.7).

Ujjayi   Type of Pranayama where the throat is slightly constricted to give a soft sound on the inhalation and exhalation. Ujjayi literally means victorious. In the Pranayama the chest is expanded like a victorious warrior's.

Upavista Konasana   *Upavista* means to sit, *Kon* means angle. Seated angle pose (Fig. 1.38).

Urdhva Dhanurasana   Upward-stretch bow pose (Fig. 1.2).

Urdhva Prasrta Padasana   Upward-stretched leg pose (Fig. 1.9).

Ustrasana   Camel pose (Fig. 1.15).

Utkatasana   Squatting posture.

Uttanasana   Forward-stretched pose (Fig. 1.5).

Vajrasana   Kneeling posture (Fig. 1.18).

Viloma   Against the grain.

Vinyasa   To go step by step, planning a sequence of postures or Pranayama.

Viparita Dandasana   Inverted rod pose (Fig. 1.42).

Virabhadrasana   Hero pose (Fig. 2.1).

Yoga   Union of the individual with the universal.

INDEX